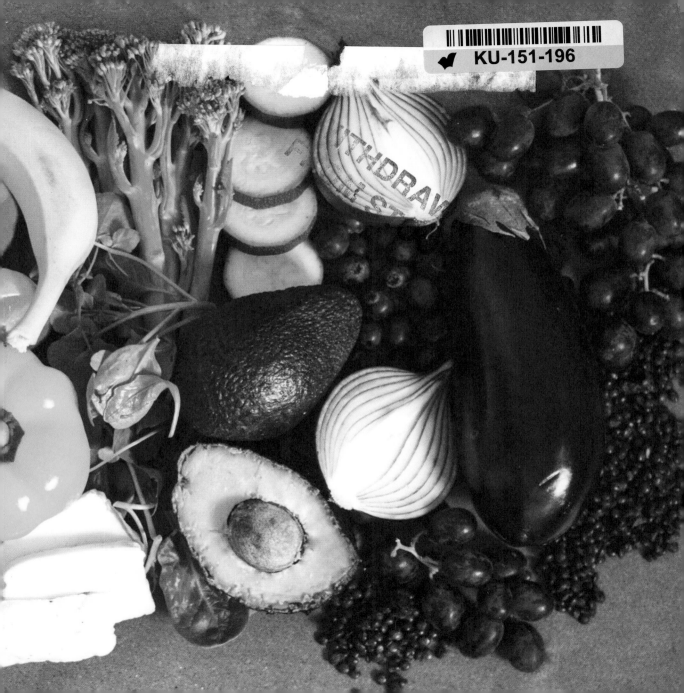

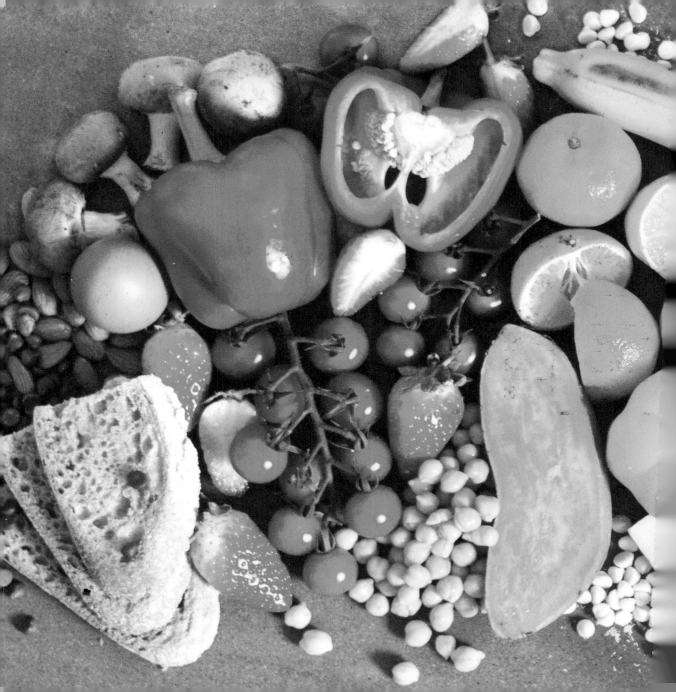

The Wellness Rebel

Plantbased Pixie is a nutritionist (MSc) (AfN), award-winning food blogger, writer and speaker. She has also been featured at many events, in various publications and on *BBC World News* and *Channel 5* as a nutritional expert.

WWW.PLANTBASED-PIXIE.COM

The Wellness Rebel

PLANTBASED PIXIE

HEAD of ZEUS

An Anima Book

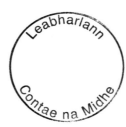

CONTENTS

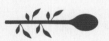

Eat 'clean'

Let's kick things off on the right foot to avoid any awkward confusion later on: this isn't a diet book, and it's not a clean-eating bible, transformation plan or miracle cure. It's about science, the science of healthy eating – in my eyes, arguably the best kind of science as it applies to us every day of our lives. This book isn't just the ramblings of yet another health blogger; I'm a trained biochemist (BSc) and nutritionist (MSc) registered with the Association for Nutrition, and I've used my blog Plantbased Pixie to chart my journey from unhealthy student to restrictive clean-eater to scientist and sceptic. I've learnt a lot since I started my blog four years ago, and I'd like to share this information with you in the hope that you find it interesting, and hopefully avoid some of the mistakes I made.

I was lucky enough to grow up in an amazing family where my mother cooked for us almost every day. While most children around me didn't regularly sit down to eat with their parents at the dinner table, my mother insisted on maintaining this German family tradition. Growing up, I ate three meals a day, every day, with my entire family, apart from school lunchtimes. Not only that, but we had a beautiful garden where my mother grew everything from apples and pears to carrots, artichokes and four different colours of tomatoes. Every summer and autumn we'd have an abundance of fresh produce that we'd pick every morning, which was both a blessing – nothing beats picking an apple straight off the tree and taking a bite – and a curse – having to eat green beans twice a day for weeks on end because we had planted too many. I was even allowed to bring my own packed lunch to school (made by my mum) years before anyone else in my year because my mother was concerned about the standard of the food. On the one hand, this was a very caring gesture, but on the flipside, maybe it was a little controlling. Control often seems to be a strong contributing factor when it comes to disordered attitudes and behaviours around food – something I was later to discover for myself.

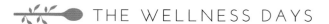 THE WELLNESS DAYS

I was an incredibly shy child, and being thrown into the new environment of university took my shyness to a new level. I turned to frozen ready meals in an attempt to both avoid cooking in the kitchen around strangers who might criticise me, and to control my food and calorie intake. University brought out all the anxiety around food that had been building for some time, and fitted in well with my perfectionism and an inherent fear of failure that had followed me around for as long as I could remember.

I knew this wasn't the healthiest way to eat, but my shyness won over my desire to be healthier. It wasn't until I had a blood test in my second year of uni, which revealed I had high cholesterol, that something switched. My grandmother had very high cholesterol and type 2 diabetes, and my father's cholesterol was dangerously high, too, which led him to start taking statins (drugs that help to keep cholesterol levels under control). As a result, it was suspected that my high cholesterol was due to familial hypercholesterolaemia, a genetic condition affecting one in 250 individuals in the UK [1], and which I had possibly inherited from my father – thanks, Dad!

I was only 19 at the time, which is very young to start taking statins, so I was given a year to make some lifestyle changes if I wanted to, but was warned that if my condition was genetic any changes would likely only have minimal effect. Naturally, I turned to Dr Google where I was bombarded with the faces and blogs of wellness 'gurus' who had faced health scares, changed their diet and seen massive success. They were beautiful, thin, happy, glowing, and promoted health rather than restriction, though they also seemed to be cutting out a variety of food groups. Naturally, I couldn't resist the charisma, and I fell for it completely. I flitted from one blogger's ideas to the next, first cutting out all refined sugar and eating more paleo-style, then going vegetarian, then full-on vegan, gluten-free, refined-sugar-free and soy-free. Basically, if there was a diet to be tried, I probably tried it.

It was at this point that I started sharing my food on Instagram as a personal food diary, and following many other accounts who ate the same way I did in order to gain inspiration on what to eat now that so many food groups were off the menu. I'll admit I went into it completely unprepared, but reassured by the many people I found online who were doing the same thing. And I'll also admit that in some ways these diets did help. On the one hand, I went to have another blood test a year later and my cholesterol was – and has since stayed – at a borderline normal/almost high level, but on the other hand, I was probably the most boring student you could imagine. My life had started to completely revolve around eating: I didn't have much of a social life, I avoided going out for meals with friends, and going home to visit my parents was an exercise in tolerance for all parties involved. My relationship with food, although appearing healthy on the outside, was definitely not ideal, and the more food groups I cut out to make my diet 'cleaner', the more anxious I became. Ironically, as my social life dwindled, my online social circle increased, thanks partly to Instagram, but also thanks to starting a blog to share my recipes, in classic wellness blogger fashion.

All these factors – food anxiety, unnecessary restriction, lack of social life, obsession with purity of ingredients – are the hallmarks of orthorexia. Orthorexia nervosa is a form of disordered eating categorised by an unhealthy, potentially dangerous obsession with eating healthily. It's an as-yet-unrecognised eating disorder that's well known in the media and with a growing body of research. I'm happy to stand up now and say, 'I had orthorexia', and let me tell you, it was not fun. And, because it's under the guise of trying to be healthy, people are much less likely to pick up on it; in fact, they're more likely to encourage you, because trying to be healthy is seen as a good thing. Which, of course, it is, but not when it causes psychological or physical damage. Despite seeming super healthy, I still didn't have amazing skin (still don't, seems to be something I'm cursed with), still wasn't happy with the way I looked and often felt tired and run-down. I never had blood tests to confirm it, but it was likely due to low iron or B12 levels from my 'super healthy' diet.

FROM WELLNESS TO REBEL

I'm happy to look back now and say 'I had orthorexia'.

After finishing uni, I used all the savings I had accumulated from three years of tutoring and scholarships and went travelling for a year. During this time, I had the opportunity to experience an amazing range of cultures. I threw myself right in at the deep end by starting my travels in India. Immediately, I was faced with a conundrum: are they using ghee (an animal product) or coconut oil in this? And you know what I did? I didn't ask, I just ate. For me, an integral part of experiencing another culture is the food, and on the diet I was following that just wasn't possible – I would be missing out on so much. When my dietary choices conflicted with my wanderlust and desire to experience the unknown, I let go and became more flexible. Temporarily. You didn't think it would really be that simple, did you!

After India, the ghee conundrum and the best food I'd ever had in my life, I spent several months in South-East Asia following the typical backpacker trail, eating pad Thai with eggs in Thailand, pho with beef in Vietnam and stir-fried vegetables with oyster sauce pretty much everywhere I went. I didn't let go completely though; whenever I took cooking classes, I made sure they were me-friendly before I went, and even had a one-to-one session with a very old Vietnamese lady who taught me how to make the best veggie pho from scratch. She gave me a piece of paper and a pencil, then expected me to write and cook with her at the same time. It was incredible.

Being SCARED of eating particular foods is not the basis for a healthy relationship with food

I still remember the turning point, the lightbulb moment where I thought to myself 'What the hell am I doing with these people?'

Next, I headed to Australia where it instantly became really easy to go back to my restrictive ways. The huge wellness culture on the east coast was a double-edged sword. I became friendly with other health bloggers and worked in an independent health food shop. I had a great time there, but being surrounded by people (both bloggers and shop customers) who were even more intensely into wellness than I was didn't help.

I still remember the exact turning point. The lightbulb moment that kickstarted everything. I was living in Melbourne, sitting in the car with some other health bloggers, when one of them stated she would never dream of vaccinating her future children. Something snapped inside me, and I thought to myself 'I'm a scientist; what the hell am I doing with these people?' I went home that day and stumbled across the online sceptical community, then devoured every fully referenced bit of information I could find. Slowly, as I read more, I began to question what these wellness gurus were saying, and when I compared their food philosophies and advice with the science, it just didn't match up. From that point onwards, every fad and unscientific principle fell by the wayside, one by one, in the face of evidence.

To this day, I have no regrets in deviating from this restrictive set of rules. I gave myself the opportunity to enjoy food, not just see it as a set of macro- and micronutrients or as a barrier to my health goals. Partly thanks to this, that year of travelling was truly the best year of my life.

Broadly speaking, if I had to use a word to describe the way I eat it would be 'plant based', partly because the definition varies widely depending on who you ask. Some fervently believe it is equivalent to a vegan diet (i.e. no animal products) without the heavily processed food, and this is probably why there have been several instances where people have been confused (and even, on occasion, become angry) when they see me eating eggs for brunch. I would like to point out that I never truly identified as vegan because my reason for eating a diet free from animal products was purely selfish, not for any selfless environmental or ethical reasons. I feel this is important to mention because it therefore means I don't directly blame veganism for my disordered behaviours. My inability to match my diet to my social life was part of the problem, but would have occurred even if I had chosen a paleo diet over a vegan diet – any such restrictive behaviours would have likely done the same. If veganism was my way in, then social media was my constant enabler and bad influence.

In the scientific literature, you can find studies on plant-based diets that range from 100% plants to only 66%. And so, as a trained scientist and nutritionist, when I talk about a 'plant-based' diet, what I mean is a diet based on plants but not necessarily solely consisting of plants. What I love about this is that it makes it accessible to pretty much everyone. Eating 100% plants is not always desirable or feasible, or even recommended, but 66% plants? That's much more manageable and much less daunting while also providing amazing health benefits.

PIXIE TIP
'Plantbased' doesn't necessarily mean 'vegan'. It can be anything from 66% to 100% plants.

BALANCE, NOT RESTRICTION

The word balance is thrown around a lot among health bloggers, but I really do believe my diet to be balanced now, because I don't pose any unnecessary restrictions on myself. I don't have any off-limits foods. I eat intuitively, and it varies day to day. By no means was that an overnight switch, though; it took many months of fighting the orthorexic/diet culture part of my brain to get to where I am now. Many bloggers claim their way of eating is 'not a diet, it's a lifestyle' and in the same breath go on to talk about food rules, staying on track and what to do when we fall off the wagon. Diets have rules that are followed; diets are started and adhered to then fail in endless cycles. Diets don't work.

A lifestyle has no rules; we can't fall off the wagon because there was no wagon to begin with. There is no need to 'stay on track during the holidays' because real life with all its variation and flaws is the track and we're always on it. We find this so hard to imagine and it sounds too good to be true because we're constantly bombarded with headlines and advice about which foods we should be avoiding and which we must eat. Just because a food is branded as 'healthy' does not make it compulsory for consumption. For example, I really hate raw kale – I could be starving on a desert island and I'd still rather eat sand – but if you enjoy it, then eat away.

I don't believe in 'healthy' and 'unhealthy' foods. Food is not healthy; food is nutritious, and if we eat nutritious foods we will (hopefully) be healthy. Similarly, foods are not 'good' or 'bad', but those words can be used to describe an overall eating pattern. In the same way that one salad won't compensate for a lifetime of unhealthy eating, one bar of chocolate won't negate a lifetime of healthy eating. I have a real issue with the language we use to describe our food and our ways of eating, and I don't feel this is something that has been talked about enough. 'Clean', 'guilt-free', 'healthy', 'good', 'real'. . . these are descriptive words that attach a moral compass to the way we eat and carry inherent judgement, pretentiousness and elitism. If I say I 'eat clean', does that make your food 'dirty'? If I call my dessert 'guilt-free', does that mean you should feel guilty for eating yours? No. Just no. Even though these opposites – 'dirty', 'guilty' – aren't always used, they are still implied, which makes them even worse. They worm their way into our subconscious, affecting our self-perception and self-worth without being able to obviously pin them down. Food is wonderful, delicious, beautiful, inviting, appetising. . . but never dirty and it should never come with feelings of guilt. No one way of eating makes a person superior to any other.

Everything is chemicals. Everything you eat and breathe is made of chemicals

Orthorexia may not sound too serious, but it has the potential to become extremely dangerous both psychologically and physically, leading to deficiencies and malnutrition. The 'clean eating' movement has encountered a considerable backlash from scientists and the public alike for its unfounded policies on restriction, endless spouting of pseudoscience, harmful use of language around food and its potential role in the development of orthorexia. From my own experiences in the wellness/clean eating world, I encountered plenty of anecdotal evidence to suggest this community, which thrives on Instagram, played a role in the development and maintenance of orthorexic tendencies. I even went on to conduct my own research, funded by the university I was at (UCL), approved by the ethics board and supervised by both a professor in nutrition and a research associate in behaviour change psychology. I determined that there was a relationship between orthorexia and social media use, with around 90% of participants showing orthorexic tendencies. That's scarily high. Now that's not to say that Instagram is inherently dangerous; it can be an incredibly inspiring place that can create lasting friendships – I met my best friends on Instagram! – but for those at risk and exposed to the wrong influences, it has the potential to lead to unhealthy attitudes towards food. I fully admit that I was one of them and acknowledging that is an important step towards using Instagram in a safe way. Instagram is great but please enjoy responsibly.

Part of the reason this clean eating movement is considered responsible for the rise of orthorexia and the reason for the backlash that followed a few years later, is the extremely unregulated nature of the information. If you look at pretty much any of the major players in the clean eating/wellness movement, you can find misinformation and pseudoscience aplenty, whether it's making gluten public enemy number one, a serious lack of understanding of the body's pH-balancing system or promoting ridiculous 'detoxing' and 'cleansing' practices. These wellness pioneers, even if well-meaning, have gained the trust of

Instagram can create lasting friendships, but can also lead to unhealthy attitudes towards food.

millions, armed only with good looks, pretty plates of food and good marketing strategies, despite often having a complete lack of nutritional qualifications. I have seen the consequences of their preaching first hand in my clients, some of who can trace back their food anxieties to specific individuals on social media. Their words and advice are simply accepted, never questioned . . . until recently.

It's okay to make mistakes, to admit to being in the wrong, to change and improve based on evidence. That's good scientific practice and I think we all need to be a little more sceptical and a little more scientific. I freely admit I made mistakes: I fell for pretty much every nugget of pseudoscience handed to me by wellness bloggers, including (but not limited to) cutting out endless food groups from my diet, believing I needed 'superfood' powders to be healthy, thinking refined sugar is toxic, not eating gluten, juicing for health, feeling the need to 'detox' my body and even doing week-long raw vegan 'cleanses'. I attached a moral compass to food. I'm not perfect, but I've learnt from these mistakes; I've taken on board new evidence and improved my understanding of nutrition and health. I've definitely made some enemies of those who were not fans of me calling them out on their fearmongering, but I believe if you haven't pissed off a few people along the way and caused a little controversy, then you haven't really achieved something new and exciting. To me, it's a sign I'm doing something right. I'm now going to help you do the same using the tools at my disposal – scientific evidence, beautiful and delicious food and a dash of sarcasm.

Each chapter in this book is going to tackle a common nutritional myth that has plagued both the wellness industry and mainstream media – everything from gluten and raw food to detoxing and superfoods. I'm going to tackle each one with the real science behind the myth, separating fact from fiction, and show you how to put this information into practice in the form of delicious, no-BS, fad-free recipes. Are you ready? Let's dive in . . .

PIXIE TIP
Every chapter in this book tackles a particular nutrition myth, but I recommend reading chapter 2 first to get the basics covered!

Food is wonderful, delicious, beautiful, inviting, appetising...
BUT NEVER DIRTY, and should never come with feelings of GUILT

Eat 'real' food

BASIC NUTRITION BIOCHEMISTRY

To be able to cut through the bullshit and recognise what might or might not be true online, having a basic understanding of nutrition biochemistry is crucial. My goal isn't to overwhelm you with complicated scientific jargon, but to go through the basics you need to know.

The composition of the food we eat can be broadly categorised into macronutrients and micronutrients. Macronutrients are required in large amounts in the diet (think quantities in grams), whereas micronutrients are necessary only in small amounts (milligrams or smaller). Macronutrients include carbohydrates (and fibre), fats and protein. Micronutrients include vitamins and minerals.

 CARBOHYDRATES

Carbohydrate literally means 'hydrated carbons', i.e. carbon atoms with water attached, so they consist of only carbon, hydrogen and oxygen atoms. Although carbohydrates are argued by some to be 'non-essential', they are the body's preferred fuel source. Common sources of carbohydrates in the diet include grains, beans, non-leafy vegetables, potatoes and sugar.

Carbohydrates can be further divided into two main groups: simple and complex carbohydrates. Simple carbs are just that – simpler, smaller structures – and so are more quickly digested by the body, whereas complex carbohydrates are more slowly digested, which is why they are considered slower releasing sources of energy.

Simple carbohydrates are monosaccharides or disaccharides. No need to be put off by big words; 'mono-' means one, 'di-' means two, and saccharide is simply a scientific word for sugar. So, a monosaccharide is a single sugar (e.g. glucose, fructose and galactose), and a disaccharide is two single sugars joined together to make a double sugar (e.g. sucrose and lactose).

PIXIE TIP
Come back to this chapter whenever you need reminding!

Glucose can be found in fruits, vegetables, grains and legumes. It is also found in grains as long chains of starch (which we'll come to in a sec) and as the disaccharide sucrose in granulated sugars and liquid sweeteners. It tends to be used as immediate fuel, or is stored as glycogen in your muscles and liver.

Fructose can be found in fruits and vegetables or as the disaccharide sucrose. If you hadn't already guessed, sucrose is what we commonly refer to as 'sugar'.

Sucrose is one glucose and one fructose molecule joined together. When you eat sucrose, an enzyme splits it into glucose and fructose. The main difference between glucose and fructose is that glucose is a 6-membered ring whereas fructose is a 5-membered ring, which means they behave differently in the body and have different metabolic rates. Glucose is metabolised throughout the body, whereas fructose is almost completely metabolised in the liver.

Remember the equation for respiration you probably learnt (and then forgot) in GCSE biology?

$$GLUCOSE + OXYGEN \longrightarrow WATER + CARBON\ DIOXIDE + ENERGY$$

This is the equation we learn to show how the body uses food for energy, and also explains why we breathe in oxygen, breathe out carbon dioxide and lose water in urine and sweat. Of course, it's not actually as simple as this, but it shows the importance of glucose. Every cell in your body has transporters to take up glucose from the blood or surroundings into the cell to use for energy. In particular, your brain relies on glucose as its energy source as it cannot directly use fats or protein for energy.

When we say 'blood sugar', what we mean is blood glucose levels. Insulin is released in response to glucose but not fructose consumption, and it helps signal to your cells to take up the glucose in the blood and use it. So, insulin responds to elevated blood glucose (from eating food), and causes blood glucose to drop again as the glucose is used by cells for energy.

When fructose is metabolised in the liver, around 25% is converted to lactate/lactic acid (responsible for the burning sensation in your muscles during an intense workout), 30–50% is converted to glucose, around 15% is converted to glycogen and less than 1% is converted to blood triglycerides (fats).

Lactose is a disaccharide of glucose and galactose, which is found in milk, hence it's also known as milk sugar. It's digested by the enzyme lactase in the intestines, except in people with lactose intolerance, where it acts as food for gut bacteria instead, leading to uncomfortable bloating and diarrhoea symptoms.

Complex carbohydrates are polysaccharides because a single chain can contain thousands of glucose molecules all joined together. One way of thinking about it is that sugars or simple carbohydrates are beads, and complex carbohydrates are a chain of beads on a string. The beads are the energy source, so if you want to access the energy in complex carbohydrates you have to take the beads off the string one at a time, which takes a lot longer than just having a pile of loose beads.

Glycogen is a polysaccharide that is the main storage form of glucose in human cells. **Starch** is a polysaccharide that is the main form of glucose storage in plants. Although you would think they'd be interchangeable, in plants and animals they're actually bonded together differently. Glycogen is found in animals, whereas starch is found in plants. Every gram of glycogen is also bound to around 2g of water, which is where the concept of losing water weight comes from, and why people can experience dramatic weight loss at the beginning of a low-carb diet [1].

When you eat starch from plants, enzymes called amylases in your body break it down into individual glucose molecules, and these are then used as energy (see previous page) or rearranged into glycogen stores. These stores are found in the muscles and liver, and they are what you then use during movement or exercise or for energy. Liver glycogen can be broken down and used by the whole body, whereas muscle glycogen is only used by the muscles. During exercise, your muscle protein structures contract, but that requires energy, which comes from the glycogen found in muscles. It's a quick, convenient energy source. When marathon runners hit 'the wall', that's the point at which their glycogen stores run out.

PHYSICAL health
should not come at the expense of
MENTAL health

The composition of the food we eat can be broadly categorised into macronutrients and micronutrients. Macronutrients are required in large amounts in the diet whereas micronutrients are necessary only in small amounts

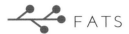 FATS

Fats are also known as triglycerides, with a structure of three fatty acid chains bound to a glycerol backbone. There are many words for fats that are often used interchangeably, for example oils, which are simply liquid fats, and lipids, which are fats but aren't necessarily triglycerides.

Fat: glycerol with 3 different chains

There are two main types of fats found in food: saturated and unsaturated fats. Unsaturated fats can be monounsaturated, polyunsaturated or trans fats. Whether a fat is saturated, monounsaturated, polyunsaturated or trans depends on the fatty acid chains.

Saturated fats have single bonds between the carbons in the fatty acid chain. Because they only have single bonds, this means there are more bonds available between carbon and hydrogen atoms, and so the carbons are 'saturated' with hydrogen. Unsaturated fats, on the other hand, have one or more double bonds between carbon atoms in the fatty acid chain. As each carbon can only form four bonds, this leaves fewer bonds to be formed between carbon and hydrogen atoms, so the carbons are 'unsaturated' (i.e. not saturated). If there is only one double bond, then it's a monounsaturated fat, and if there's more than one, it's a polyunsaturated fat.

If you look at the diagram on the previous page, this will hopefully make more sense. The first of the fatty acid chains is saturated, the second is monounsaturated and the third is polyunsaturated. These differences are important. Saturated fats have a regular structure so they can pack together tightly, which is why sources of saturated fat are often solid – for example, butter or cheese. Unsaturated fats can't pack together as tightly, so they are usually liquid – for example, olive oil.

We name unsaturated fats based on the non-acid end (i.e. the end not attached to glycerol). This end is called n-end or omega end. Hopefully a lightbulb has just gone off in your head and you're thinking of omega-3 and omega-6 fats. Both are types of polyunsaturated fatty acids (PUFA). Omega-3 fatty acids are so called because the 3rd carbon from the end is the first double-bonded carbon, whereas omega-6 fatty acids are so called because the 6th carbon from the end is the first double-bonded carbon.

The human body can make most of the types of fats it needs from other fats or raw materials. Omega-3 PUFA are essential fatty acids as they cannot be made by humans, so we have to obtain them from food. (Note: essential oils are a completely different kettle of fish; they're 'essential' as they are concentrated essences, not because we need them in some way to function.) The three types of omega-3 PUFA involved in human physiology are α-linolenic acid (ALA), eicosapentaenoic acid (EPA) and docosahexaenoic acid (DHA). ALA is found in plants, whereas EPA and DHA are commonly found in fish oils. Your body can convert ALA to EPA and DHA, but not very effectively. As such, ALA is the only omega-3 PUFA that is essential, although DHA and EPA are conditionally essential – which means they are considered essential in some conditions.

Of the omega-6 PUFA, linoleic acid, the shortest one, is the only essential fatty acid. The body can convert this to longer chain fatty acids. Sources of omega-6 include most vegetable oils, eggs, nuts and whole grains.

In general, we're very good at getting enough omega-6 fats in our diet, but less so at getting enough omega-3. You may have heard that omega-3 is anti-inflammatory while omega-6 is pro-inflammatory, but it's actually a bit more complicated than that . . . but I digress. This isn't the chapter for myth-busting!

Omega-7 and omega-9 fatty acids are monounsaturated, and are not essential as your body can make these from other fats. Olive oil, rapeseed oil, avocados (whole and oil) and macadamia nut oil are all rich sources of these.

Trans fats are also unsaturated fats, and have the double bond in a different configuration to those generally naturally found in foods – the trans rather than cis configuration. Trans fats occur in small amounts in nature, but have appeared in our diets due to food processing known as hydrogenation. This is where liquid cis-unsaturated fats such as vegetable oils are partially hydrogenated (by adding hydrogen) to make them more saturated and therefore melt at lower temperatures – think spreadable fats like margarine. During this process, the cis double bonds are broken and can be rearranged as trans double bonds.

Fat can be an energy source for the body, and can be stored during times of excess. When needed, fats are broken down to produce glycerol and fatty acids. The glycerol can then be converted into glucose by the liver, thereby becoming a source of energy, whereas fatty acids are broken down by a complex process called β-oxidation. Fats are an amazing form of energy storage by the body, much more so than glycogen, as they're more compact, don't attract water and store more energy per gram. A gram of fat stores more than 6 times as much energy as a gram of hydrated glycogen. So, as an example, if you weigh 70kg

PIXIE TIP
Omega-3 and omega-6 are the essential fatty acids that we have to obtain from our diet.

In some cases, cooking food can break down some vitamins, but in other cases it makes them easier for your body to use with 100,000kcal worth of fuel reserved as triglycerides (enough to last several weeks), this makes up around 11kg of your body weight. If this energy were stored as glycogen, your body weight would be 125kg – so 55kg more [2]! Fat is much more efficient.

Finally, a word on cholesterol, which is also technically a dietary fat. Cholesterol is an essential part of every one of your cells, and can be made by the body. Cholesterol is also the precursor to several hormones (cortisol, testosterone, oestrogen, etc.) as well as vitamin D. Technically, we don't need any cholesterol from our diet whatsoever. Plant cells do not manufacture cholesterol, so it is not found in plant foods, only in animal foods such as cheese, egg yolks, meat and fish. We'll be talking much more about cholesterol and health later on in the chapter on fats.

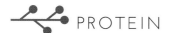 PROTEIN

Proteins are long chains of amino acids, twisted into highly complex 3D shapes that serve highly specific functions. Amino acids are the building blocks, like the beads on a chain, with several common features.

Amino acid structure

AMINO GROUP   CARBOXYL GROUP

SIDE CHAIN

All amino acids have a central carbon, an amino group (NH_2), a carboxylic acid group (COOH) – hence the name amino acid – and an R roup which is different in every single amino acid. This difference is important as it means every amino acid behaves differently, and so will cause the protein to fold differently in the final 3D structure. The sequence of amino acids dictates the final shape of a protein.

Each amino acid has a full name, a three-letter shorthand and a single-letter shorthand for when chemists are feeling really lazy. There are twenty protein-forming amino acids encoded in the human genome, and of these twenty, there are nine essential amino acids that the body can't synthesise. Every other amino acid can be created from other structures, including other amino acids, but these nine have to come from the diet. In case you're interested, the essential amino acids are: Phenylalanine, Valine, Threonine, Tryptophan, Methionine, Leucine, Isoleucine, Lysine and Histidine.

Food sources that have all nine of these in similar amounts to what our bodies need are known as complete protein sources. Most animal protein sources are complete proteins, whereas few plant sources are. Quinoa, buckwheat, soy and mycoprotein are examples of complete sources. Otherwise, you can combine plant sources to give a meal with complete protein, such as rice and beans or hummus and pita.

Branched chain amino acids (BCAAs) are what it says on the tin: amino acids with branches in their side chain. There are three in humans, valine, leucine and isoleucine, all of which are essential amino acids. These three make up around 35% of your muscle mass and promote protein synthesis, which is why they're such popular supplements. But don't think you need to supplement in order to build muscle. If you're meeting your daily protein requirements (0.8g protein per kg of body weight per day), then it's pretty certain you'll meet your BCAA requirements, as they're found in all protein-containing foods.

PIXIE TIP
You can combine foods to create a meal with complete protein, or eat them separately throughout the day!

When we eat protein, the protein chains are broken down into individual amino acids by enzymes called proteases in the stomach and small intestines. These are then small enough to be absorbed into the bloodstream and transported around the body. This is important because collagen supplements, for example, are claimed to boost collagen levels in your skin, when, in fact, they're broken down just like any other protein and then built up again into whatever your body decides it needs, and there's only a tiny chance that's actually going to be collagen. Your body doesn't absorb complete proteins; they're just too big.

Protein isn't just for building muscle – although this is a significant part of it. Some amino acids are also precursors for some neurotransmitters such as dopamine and serotonin. Proteins also act as messengers to help send signals within a cell and from cell to cell, and they act as transporters to move specific substances in and out of cells. Proteins can also be enzymes; in fact, all enzymes are proteins (although not all proteins are enzymes, of course). Enzymes are biological catalysts that speed up and facilitate reactions in the body. Without them, you'd be dead, as nothing would happen fast enough in your body. Every enzyme has a unique structure with an active site where the substrate slots in – think of Pac-Man as the enzyme with a uniquely shaped mouth that can only fit one or a small number of molecules inside. Enzymes are highly specific and won't accept anything that isn't the exact shape and size it's designed to fit.

Enzymes break the bonds between molecules in digestion (kind of funny really, proteins breaking down proteins), allowing your body to absorb the ones it needs. They also convert toxic substances into ones that are safe to excrete, and they're involved in metabolism by converting substances or adding or taking away elements of it.

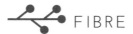 FIBRE

Fibre is the indigestible part of plant foods. It can be soluble, which dissolves in water, is easily fermented in the gut and can be prebiotic. Or it can be insoluble, which does not dissolve in water. Insoluble fibre can be either metabolically inert and have bulking action or can be fermented and prebiotic.

Fibre acts by changing the intestinal contents and altering how nutrients are absorbed. There are three primary mechanisms by which fibre acts: bulking, viscosity and fermentation. Bulking fibres absorb water as they move through the digestive system, which increases stool weight and keeps you 'going' regularly. Viscous fibres thicken up the contents of the intestine and thereby stop certain nutrients such as sugars or cholesterol from being absorbed. They can be partly fermented, fully fermented or not fermented at all. Fermentable fibres are digested by your gut bacteria (your microbiome) in the large intestines, which produce short-chain fatty acids as metabolic by-products (more on these in a bit).

Different fibres from different foods have different effects, suggesting that a variety of dietary fibres contribute to overall health. Plant foods tend to have both soluble and insoluble fibres, so they are divided into which they provide more of. Soluble fibre is particularly found in legumes, oats, rye, nuts, some fruits, broccoli, carrots, root vegetables, psyllium husk and flaxseed. Insoluble fibre is particularly found in whole grains, legumes, nuts, seeds and vegetable and fruit skins.

As a general population, we don't eat enough fibre. We should be aiming for around 30g per day to get all the benefits from it. Oh, I haven't told you about the benefits yet, have I? Here goes . . .

Dietary fibre increases food volume without increasing calorie content (so you feel full and satisfied sooner), as well as delaying gastric emptying leading to extended feelings of fullness. It also helps prevent or relieve constipation, feeds your gut microbiome and stimulates fermentation production of short-chain fatty acids. These short-chain fatty acids help stabilise blood glucose levels, regulate glucose absorption, provide food for intestinal cells (particularly butyrate), suppress cholesterol synthesis by the liver, reduce blood levels of LDL cholesterol and triglycerides, and lower the pH of the gut which helps increase absorption of minerals and stimulate production of various immune cells and components [3].

On top of that, dietary fibre is linked to reduced risk of death from cardiovascular disease [4], all types of cancer [4], infectious diseases and respiratory diseases [5]. It's also linked to reduced risk of developing type 2 diabetes [6]. So, eat your fibre!

Of course, at this point I should mention that there are some downsides to eating lots of fibre. If you increase your fibre intake too quickly, there is a risk of bloating and flatulence as your gut microbiome adjusts to the change. But considering all the benefits and the fact that we have a serious constipation problem in this country [7], I'd say the benefits outweigh the temporary risks.

MICRONUTRIENTS: VITAMINS & MINERALS

Vitamins and minerals are essential nutrients that the body needs in small amounts, ranging from a few milligrams to single micrograms (µg or 1 millionth of a gram). Although the amounts are tiny, without these vitamins and minerals our health suffers. Deficiency is not always visible straight away, sometimes it can take years of deficiency for overt symptoms to appear, and in other cases, just a matter of weeks.

There are two types of vitamins: water-soluble and fat-soluble vitamins. The water-soluble vitamins are vitamin C and the B vitamins; these dissolve in water and are not stored by the body so we need to get them from our diet every day. The fat-soluble vitamins are vitamins A, D, E and K; these dissolve in fat before being taken up into the bloodstream and are stored in the liver so they are not needed every day but still regularly in the diet.

VITAMIN	ALTERNATE NAME	FUNCTION	RDI*	FOOD SOURCES
A	Retinol/carotenoids	Immune system, vision, healthy skin	0.7mg for men 0.6mg for women	Cheese, eggs, milk, carrots, sweet potatoes, spinach, peppers
B1	Thiamine	Nervous system, unlocking the energy in food	1mg for men 0.8mg for women	Peas, fruit, eggs, whole grains
B2	Riboflavin	Healthy skin, eyes and nervous system, unlocking the energy in food	1.3mg for men 1.1mg for women	Milk, eggs, fortified breakfast cereals, rice
B3	Niacin	Healthy skin and nervous system, unlocking the energy in food	16.5mg for men 13.2mg for women	Meat, fish, wheat, eggs, milk
B5	Pantothenic acid	Unlocking the energy in food, food metabolism	17mg for men 13mg for women	Almost all meat and vegetables, whole grains

VITAMIN	ALTERNATE NAME	FUNCTION	RDI*	FOOD SOURCES
B6	Pyridoxine	Forming haemoglobin, unlocking and storing energy in carbs and protein	1.4mg for men 1.2mg for women	Poultry, fish, whole grains, eggs, vegetables, soy
B7	Biotin	Breaking down fat, cell growth	50µg for men and women	Leafy green vegetables, raw egg yolk; also made by the microbiome
B9	Folate/folic acid	Formation of red blood cells	200µg for men and women; 400µg for women if trying for a baby	Green vegetables, chickpeas and other legumes, oranges
B12	Cobalamin	Formation of red blood cells, unlocking energy in food, healthy nervous system	1.5µg for men and women	Meat, fish, eggs, cheese, milk
C	Ascorbic acid	Helping with wound healing, healthy skin, blood vessels, bones and cartilage	40mg for men and women	Oranges, broccoli, berries, peppers

VITAMIN	ALTERNATE NAME	FUNCTION	RDI*	FOOD SOURCES
D		Healthy bones, teeth and muscles	10μg for men and women	Oily fish, liver, egg yolks, fortified foods; from sunlight in summer months
E		Healthy immune system, skin and eyes	4mg for men 3mg for women	Plant oils, nuts, seeds, avocados
K		Wound healing, healthy bones	1μg per kg of body weight per day	Leafy green vegetables, vegetable oils

*RDI = recommended daily intake

Minerals are chemical elements required as essential nutrients by our bodies. They are not the same as vitamins because vitamins are complex chemical structures, whereas minerals are single elements that can be found on the periodic table.

There are five major minerals found in the human body: calcium, phosphorus, potassium, sodium and magnesium. The remaining elements in the body are called trace elements. Of particular note are iron, copper, zinc, manganese, iodine and selenium.

MINERAL	FUNCTION	RDI*	FOOD SOURCES
Potassium	Controlling fluid balance, sending electrical signals around the body	3500mg for men and women	Sweet potatoes, tomatoes, potatoes, legumes, dairy foods, seafood, bananas, chicken
Sodium	Controlling fluid balance, sending electrical signals around the body	2400mg for men and women	Table salt, seaweed, milk
Calcium	Building bones and teeth, regulating muscle contractions	700mg for men and women	Dairy foods, leafy vegetables, soy, nuts, fish where you eat the bones
Phosphorus	Building bones and teeth, releasing energy in food	550mg for men and women	Meat, dairy foods, fish, bread, brown rice, oats
Magnesium	Helping parathyroid glands function normally, obtaining energy from food	300mg for men 270mg for women	Spinach, legumes, nuts, seeds, whole grains, peanut butter, avocados
Iron	Making red blood cells	8.7mg for men 14.8mg for women (8.7mg post-menopause)	Meat, beans, nuts, leafy vegetables
Zinc	Making new cells, making enzymes, wound healing, processing carbohydrate, fat and protein in food	9.5mg for men 7mg a day for women	Meat, shellfish, dairy foods, bread, cereals
Manganese	Making and activating enzymes	1.4mg for men and women	Grains, legumes, seeds, nuts, leafy vegetables, tea, coffee

MINERAL	FUNCTION	RDI*	FOOD SOURCES
Copper	Making red and white blood cells, healthy immune system	1.2mg for men and women	Shellfish, whole grains, beans, nuts, potatoes, organ meats
Iodine	Thyroid hormones	0.14mg for men and women	Seafood, some plants but dependent on soil
Selenium	Healthy immune system, reproductive system, antioxidant function	0.075mg for men 0.06mg for women	Brazil nuts, fish, meat, eggs

*RDI = recommended daily intake

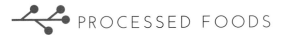 PROCESSED FOODS

The message in the wellness industry is very much a focus on good vs evil; natural foods vs processed ones. We are told that processed foods are essentially the root of all evil and we must eliminate them at all costs in order to achieve optimum health. Not only is this unrealistic (who really has time to prepare every single thing from scratch?!) but it is also not based on evidence.

If you think about it, pretty much everything is processed in some way. Cooking, chopping and freezing are all forms of processing. But I can imagine you're probably rolling your eyes at that and thinking that's not a good enough argument and fair enough. But processing food is important. It has helped reduce the presence of bacteria in our food, thereby reducing food poisoning, and it has led to foods becoming cheaper and more easily accessible to those who couldn't afford them otherwise.

Yes, it has also caused problems, let's be realistic, but we can't discount all the huge benefits food processing has offered us.

Just because something has been made in a factory doesn't make it inherently bad for you. Many 'health' products are made in factories, from raw brownies to nut butters, with one ingredient to more than ten, but it's the ingredients that contribute to how nutritious something is, not whether it's made at home or in a factory. You can make a dish at home that contains more fat or sugar or salt than the same product bought in a supermarket or you could make a dish that contains less.

To use the blanket term 'processed food' so negatively also completely fails to acknowledge the fact that many wonderfully nutritious foods are processed. Canned tomatoes and beans, bottled egg whites, packets of cooked lentils, jars of pesto . . . these are all wonderful, convenient and nutritionally dense foods. I don't deny that eating an abundance of ultra-processed foods is probably not a great idea, but there's no need to say we have to eliminate all processed foods entirely. We should be promoting balance, moderation and eating a variety of foods, not making sweeping statements about exclusion and restriction.

I've seen wellness bloggers and authors say things like, 'These foods are so processed that by the time they reach your plate it's hard for your body to even recognise them'. How do you think your body works? Do you think you eat a meal and your body goes, 'Mmm, avocado and eggs'. It does not. Your body recognises carbohydrate chains, fat, proteins to degrade, vitamins and minerals. It recognises bonds between molecules that it needs to break down. It doesn't 'know' where they came from, it just does its job turning food into energy. Stop romanticising how the body works.

Everything you eat and breathe is made of chemicals. Oxygen is a chemical; water is a chemical; vitamin C is a chemical. Even something as harmless and loved as vitamin C can sound scary when you call it E300 instead. Using the term 'chemicals' to mean something negative and unhealthy is misinformed

PIXIE TIP
Don't dismiss foods just because they are 'processed' – in some cases they can be the best time-savers and just as nutritious.

The concept of 'real food' does not exist

and fearmongering. Just because you can't pronounce something or don't recognise it, doesn't make it bad for you; basing your diet on your knowledge of chemistry is incredibly reductionist and backwards. I'll bet you can pronounce cyanide easily, but that doesn't make it sensible for you to eat. I'll also bet you can't pronounce a lot of the antioxidants and enzymes naturally found in plants (peroxiredoxin or phenylenediamine anyone?), yet they're fine to eat. A subset of the population is terrified at the prospect of formaldehyde, yet your body produces it all the time as part of its natural metabolism. Being afraid of foods, or even worse, instilling these fears in others, is incredibly damaging.

Artificial doesn't equal bad, and natural doesn't equal good. It's not that simple. It's another example of not just how elitist the wellness industry is, but also how much it relies on nostalgia. There's always a cry for the 'good old days' where everything was made from scratch and we were all at 'peak health'. Except we weren't. We also had high infant mortality rates, had high rates of preventable communicable disease, starved during the winter due to a lack of fresh local produce, and women were chained to the kitchen all day to feed their families. Thanks to science, we now have an abundant food supply, have foods with longer shelf lives to reduce waste, and we can spend our time doing other things like having a career and a social life (should we so choose) instead of spending all day in the kitchen making stocks, sauces and pastries. Be thankful for science and progress; they're the reason we now have exotic and new ingredients like quinoa and protein powders, and the reason we are living longer than ever before.

The concept of 'real food' does not exist. This attitude of demonising convenience and anything artificial or not produced on a farm is not only elitist and discriminating, but is also damaging. Shaming people into eating healthily is not right, and doesn't work, in the same way that weight stigma and shaming people into losing weight doesn't work [8]. And neither does judging people for their food choices. When you see a stranger eating something you wouldn't choose yourself, for whatever reason, you know nothing of their social, financial, emotional or physical situation. You have no right to judge them for what they are eating. What someone chooses to eat and chooses not to eat are personal decisions, particularly if they are someone who has struggled with their body and their relationship with food. And let's face it, that's a huge percentage of the population, especially in the UK. Surveys regularly show that people in the UK, especially women, have one of the lowest body confidence scores in the world [9], and up to 90% of British adult women feel body-image anxiety [10].

Our use of moral language around food needs to change. Nutrition isn't black and white, there is no 'good' and 'bad', no 'processed' and 'unprocessed'; it all lies on a continuous spectrum, with some foods being more nutritious than others, and some more processed than others. The idea of all processed foods being bad and anything natural being good is just one of the many myths that have been perpetuated by the wellness industry. Let's look at a few more . . .

Nutrition isn't black and white, there is no 'good' and 'bad', no 'processed' and 'unprocessed'; it all lies on a continuous spectrum

Gluten

THE GLUTEN MYTH

American television host Jimmy Kimmel, in one of his famous videos, went out on to the streets of America and asked people if they ate gluten. Many said no. He then asked these people, 'What is gluten?'. They didn't know! Honestly, I find it baffling that people would avoid something without even knowing what it is.

So, let's talk gluten.

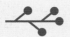 WHAT EVEN IS GLUTEN?

Gluten is a group of proteins, composed of mainly gliadin and glutenin. If you suffer from coeliac disease your body produces an autoimmune reaction to the gliadin part of the gluten protein (in most cases, at least), but more on that later. For the vast majority of the population who don't have coeliac disease, the body simply digests gluten just like any other protein. Gluten is found in grains like wheat, spelt, barley and rye. It is also sometimes added to packaged food to improve texture and flavour and to retain moisture.

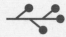 WHAT DOES IT DO?

Gluten is a group of proteins that give dough elasticity.

Gluten gives elasticity to dough, helps it keep its shape and gives a chewy texture. The name comes from its glue-like properties. The glutenin molecules cross-link to form a network attached to gliadin and create the stringiness and thickness to dough. The more gluten is worked and developed, the chewier the texture. The gluten network also traps carbon dioxide, helping bread to rise. That's why recipes say to knead dough for a certain length of time. Bread doughs have high gluten strength, whereas pastry tends to be lower in gluten.

If you compare wheat-based bread to gluten-free bread, the wheat-based loaves have a better rise, whereas the gluten-free ones are less springy and more brittle [1]. The textures are quite different. I think I've only once had gluten-free bread that tasted good, and it was drowning in avocado, so that's probably not a reliable comparison. Bread is wonderful, and using gluten makes baking so much easier. So why would you avoid it out of choice?

I love bread. To me, it is one of the great joys in life. From the therapeutic kneading of the dough, to the hollow sound it produces when you tap the base. There's crusty baguette that you tear apart with your hands, soft ciabatta that feels like holding a pillow, the wonderful smell of sourdough. . . and that's not even mentioning the eating part. That contrast of crust that works your teeth and soft, holey insides. The variety of flavours available simply by changing flours or enriching the dough with sugar or butter. And don't even get me started on garlic bread. Bread is the perfect base for any meal of the day, whether it's topped with avocado and eggs for breakfast, seals a variety of textures and flavours into a sandwich for lunch or is dipped into shakshuka or soup for dinner. No one food encompasses the idea of comfort food the way bread does. Show me a person who doesn't have wonderful bread-related memories and I'll show you someone who hasn't lived. Bread is a hug in food form. Bread is happiness. I wouldn't want to live without bread.

The history of human culture is tied to the history of bread. Most cultures have some form of bread as a staple component of the diet. It helps that it's pretty cheap too, as well as a great source of energy (or calories).

No food encompasses the idea of comfort the way bread does.

In the last couple of years, there has been a growing number of people going gluten-free for a variety of reasons. Firstly, we have a group of wellness bloggers who have either shunned gluten for 'health reasons' or proclaim it to be terribly bad for you, spouting nutribollocks like 'gluten is like sandpaper for the gut'. That, along with the rise in paleo advocates, has likely contributed to an increase in the number of people going gluten-free. Secondly, gluten has become a convenient scapegoat to blame for a whole host of vague, non-specific symptoms, thereby making it a more socially-acceptable form of self-imposed restriction and rigid dietary control. Thirdly, there is an increased awareness and better diagnosis of coeliac disease. I'm going to mainly focus on the first two.

But first, let's briefly touch on coeliac disease, as I think it's important to mention the seriousness of this condition, and how different this is to someone simply deciding to cut out gluten for 'health reasons'.

COELIAC DISEASE AND WHEAT ALLERGY, AKA LEGITIMATE REASONS FOR NOT EATING GLUTEN

Coeliac disease is an autoimmune condition, in which the immune system mistakes a component of gluten proteins for a threat and attacks it. This causes an inflammatory reaction in the small intestine, which can lead to damage to the gut lining, disrupting the absorption of nutrients. Malabsorption is one of the common symptoms of coeliac disease, along with diarrhoea, abdominal pain, bloating, wind, indigestion, constipation, fatigue (due to malabsorption resulting in anaemia) and weight loss (again due to malabsorption of nutrients).

As a result, the only way to manage it is by completely eliminating gluten from the diet. The current incidence in the UK is reported to be around 1%, but the true figure is likely to be higher than this due to underdiagnosis [2]. It's important to note that coeliac disease can only be diagnosed if the person is eating gluten when being tested.

Wheat allergy, on the other hand, is an allergic reaction resulting from exposure to wheat proteins, either by contact or ingestion. Over twenty different causes have been identified, so gluten isn't necessarily the culprit. Usually, it's very specific. Symptoms can include eczema, hives, abdominal pain, nausea and vomiting. Management simply involves eliminating wheat and, in some cases, all gluten-containing grains, although this depends on the exact protein that causes the allergy.

It goes without saying that if you think you have coeliac disease or a wheat allergy, please get this properly diagnosed by a medical professional. Please don't self-diagnose.

Right, now that I'm done with these two medical conditions, let's talk about the more interesting and vague non-coeliac gluten sensitivity (NCGS).

NON-COELIAC GLUTEN SENSITIVITY

In 2011, NCGS was defined as 'a non-allergenic and non-autoimmune condition in which the consumption of gluten can lead to symptoms similar to those seen in coeliac disease' [3]. Coeliac disease isn't seen as controversial, but NCGS is, and it's still debated as to whether it actually exists or not.

Of those with NCGS self-diagnosis, there are likely to be some who experience a nocebo effect. This is similar to the placebo effect but with negative outcomes instead of positive ones. So, an individual may read a blog saying gluten is the devil, and then next time they eat gluten they expect to experience symptoms, so they appear. The mind is incredibly powerful in this way. Aside from nocebo effect, individuals may have irritable bowel syndrome (and don't forget, many foods can trigger IBS), undiagnosed coeliac disease, or an intolerance to foods that have coincidentally also been excluded from the diet. Some may be hypochondriacs (sorry) and some may possibly have actual NCGS (estimated at possibly 3% of the population). So NCGS itself could be similar to coeliac disease but without the autoimmune response, or like IBS in terms of intestinal mobility issues or it could be similar to food allergies. But this means there may be multiple mechanisms by which it occurs, which confuses the diagnostic criteria and methods of diagnosis. It's hard to tell due to widespread self-diagnosis and self-treatment. This confusion has led to researchers suggesting a range of terms to describe this, including non-coeliac wheat sensitivity, wheat protein sensitivity, or non-coeliac gluten sensitivity.

It's not as simple as cutting out gluten, seeing symptoms improve and therefore assuming the cause of any issues must be gluten. Why, you ask? Well, this is because gluten is found in so many ingredients and foods, and cutting out something as staple as gluten-containing grains involves a pretty large shift in the diet. There are also so many different things individuals can replace these gluten-containing foods with, and any one of these foods could be playing a role. There are simply too many changes to the diet to be able to determine that gluten is the problem. What about other ingredients commonly found in gluten-containing foods? What if the macronutrient ratio in the diet is shifted? What if an individual replaces gluten-containing foods with a whole host of extra fruits and vegetables? So many variables! All these things could be having an effect. We simply can't say that the problem is gluten, but it's become a convenient scapegoat for people to latch on to, so they blame the gluten. I don't mean to be

PIXIE TIP
If you think you have a problem with gluten, try eating slower and chewing more, before considering an elimination diet.

condescending – it's very easy to see how this simple conclusion can be drawn – but it's only once you dig deeper and look at it with a more critical scientific eye that you start to see all the other factors that could easily play a role. It's also important to remember that a likely scenario is that when someone presents with gastric issues, their friend says, 'Oh hey, it might be gluten; I cut it out and felt better. Give it a try!', so that person then starts restricting foods with a preconceived idea of what the problem could be, and any positive outcome will be immediately attributed to absence of gluten, because it's at the forefront of the mind. Funny how the mind works.

Before gluten sensitivity can be diagnosed, it's important to exclude coeliac disease and other organic diseases. It's also much more complex than simply cutting out gluten and seeing what happens. It needs a personalised, evidence-based approach that involves finding out more about the person's diet and lifestyle, identifying a range of possible dietary triggers, and blinded challenges to avoid bias. Often if someone experiences bloating after eating a large bowl of, say, pasta, the problem isn't the pasta itself. Often the bloating is caused by overeating, eating too quickly, or not chewing properly.

We can't say for sure whether NCGS exists or not, but saying that it doesn't isn't exactly going to help those people who still have unexplained symptoms, and it isn't going to make them feel better about themselves.

One way to determine if it exists is to test using blinded exposure. This has been tried before; individuals who self-diagnosed with NCGS were exposed to gluten in a blind crossover study. Many observed no reaction to gluten, which suggests gluten wasn't actually the problem, they just thought it was [4]. But some did respond to a low FODMAP diet, which includes eliminating major sources of gluten such as wheat, which is important to note.

I've mentioned FODMAPs a few times now, so what are they? FODMAP stands for fermentable oligo-, di-, monosaccharides and polyols. These are poorly absorbed, short-chain carbohydrates, which are found in a whole host of foods including onions, garlic, figs and many types of beans. A low FODMAP diet has been shown to be incredibly effective for around 70–75% of IBS sufferers [5], but as it's such a restrictive diet, it should always be done under the supervision of a specialist dietitian and shouldn't be followed long-term. Under supervision, it is usually strictly followed for around four to six weeks, and then, if symptoms are resolved, foods are systematically reintroduced to try to incorporate as much variety as possible in the diet without producing symptoms.

I don't want the low FODMAP diet to become the new weight-loss fad, so here's a quick deterrent: a low FODMAP diet reduces the abundance of gut bacteria, whereas a higher FODMAP diet is associated with promoting the growth of beneficial bacteria [5]. I can't stress just how important this is – your gut bacteria have a huge influence on your wellbeing and research indicates that having a more diverse gut microbiome is a key marker of gut health.

> A gluten-free diet is not necessarily healthier than one that contains gluten.

Less than 5% of the population have a legitimate problem with gluten, and yet according to the BBC an estimated 8.5 million people in the UK say they have gone gluten-free. This means there is a huge number of people who are excluding gluten unnecessarily.

HOW HEALTHY IS A GLUTEN-FREE DIET?

The craze for gluten-free products has improved the lives of those with coeliac disease, who are more catered for now than ever before. Aside from those with genuine allergies, coeliac disease and IBS, there are plenty of individuals who are going gluten-free to either treat a host of vague symptoms like 'brain fog' or simply because they've been told it's healthier. But is a gluten-free diet even healthier? Not necessarily.

Gluten-free versions of common foods often have a range of additional ingredients to compensate for the lack of gluten and to recreate the texture and mouthfeel of gluten-containing foods. This means these alternatives can be higher in added sugars or fats. Gluten-free diets, both in the short and long term, have been found to be lower in calcium, iron, folate, thiamine, niacin, B12 and fibre [6, 7, 8]. It's worth noting though, that naturally gluten-free grains such as amaranth, quinoa and buckwheat have great nutritional profiles, and are recommended alternatives to gluten-containing grains [9].

Gluten-containing grains such as wheat and barley tend to be high in fibre, and this is important as fibre affects your gut bacteria. A gluten-free diet has been linked to a reduction in beneficial bacteria populations in the gut, which may also influence the immune function of these gut bacteria [10].

In addition to not necessarily being healthier, there's also the issue of cost. Here in the UK, gluten-free foods are less widely available and often considerably more expensive than their standard counterparts [11]. So the kind of person who goes gluten-free out of choice is also likely the kind of person for whom this extra cost is not an issue as it won't significantly impact their finances – the so-called 'worried well'. The gluten-free trend is a classic example of the elitism of the wellness industry – if it's more expensive, it's more desirable, because it discriminates and shows that you can afford to spend more money on something more expensive, even though you don't really need to. This is a theme you'll be seeing throughout this book, and one of the key reasons why I'm not a fan of the wellness industry (as if the title wasn't obvious enough . . .).

Beyond this, there are other factors to consider, such as the social implications of a gluten-free diet. Every coeliac I've ever met laments the lack of options when they go out to eat and the awkwardness of asking others to accommodate their needs at dinner parties and special occasions. They don't understand why anyone would willingly subject themselves to that and I see their point.

As a side note, can I just say, that for an industry obsessed with 'natural' products, the shunning of something as natural as gluten in wellness makes no sense to me. It is possible that we are eating more gluten than we generally realise, especially as it's often added to packaged foods to increase the springiness and improve texture. It's also not declared on food packaging. What's not true is that we're now eating more gluten because we have modified wheat to make it contain more gluten. Sure, we've improved wheat to make it shorter, sturdier and higher yield (all good things I'm sure you'd agree), but we haven't made it more 'gluten-dense'. And if you're eating bread that has been left to rise naturally, then there's far less chance of having gluten added.

A key to gut health, and therefore overall health, is having a varied diet with a whole range of foods. So why not let that include grains and gluten? (Unless you have coeliac disease in which case please don't.) It'll make your social life easier, it'll make you happier (carbs make you happy!) and it'll mean you can try all the delicious gluten-containing and gluten-free recipes in this chapter. I've based my decision of grain purely on taste, texture and ease, not on whether it contains gluten or not.

A key to gut health, and therefore overall health, is having a varied diet.

The gluten-free trend is a classic example of the elitism of the wellness industry - if it's more expensive, it's more desirable, because it discriminates and shows that you can afford to spend money on something more expensive, even though you don't really need to

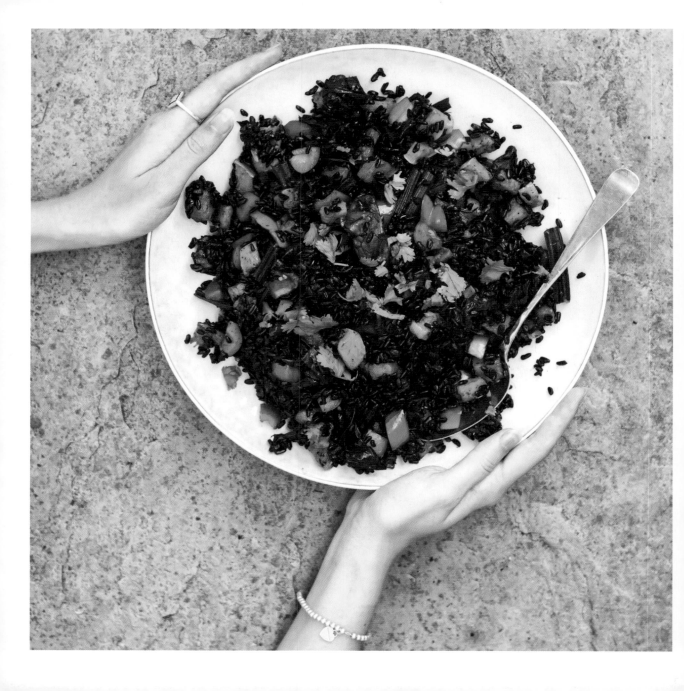

BLACK RICE WITH BUTTERNUT SQUASH AND CHARD

SERVES 4-6

- 250g black rice
- 1 tbsp soy sauce
- ½ lemon, juiced
- 400g butternut squash, peeled and cubed
- Olive oil
- Salt and pepper
- 150g rainbow chard, roughly chopped
- 1 red pepper, cubed
- Fresh coriander leaves, to serve

Black rice, like all rice, is naturally gluten-free and delicious. Black rice has the mildest effect on blood sugar levels, so if you love your grains but find they don't always work for you, this might be the one to try. Me? I just love the colour!

Preheat the oven to 200°C fan/220°C conventional/gas mark 7.

Cook the rice in boiling water with the soy sauce and lemon juice according to the packet instructions, but for 1 minute less than stated.

Spread the butternut squash over a baking tray, drizzle with olive oil and season with salt and pepper. Roast in the oven for around 30 minutes, until soft.

When the rice is cooked, remove from the heat, drain any remaining water and stir in the chard. Leave the lid on for another 5 minutes.

Add the butternut squash and red pepper to the rice, stir and season to taste.

Serve in a big bowl with fresh coriander on top.

TIP If you're a meat-eater, this recipe would also taste great with chicken.

BREAKFAST IN BREAD

SERVES 1 HUNGRY
PERSON

- 1 small sourdough loaf
- 20g spinach leaves
- 80g tomatoes, sliced
- 50g white or chestnut
  mushrooms, sliced
- 1 medium egg, separated
- Salt and pepper
- 50g grated cheddar cheese

I love a good food pun. I saw something like this in a viral video on social media around the time I was recipe testing and knew straight away this was something I needed to make. I just love bread. To avoid wasting any bread, you can turn the scooped out insides into croutons!

Preheat the oven to 180°C fan/200°C conventional/gas mark 6. Cut the top off the loaf and hollow it out.

Lay the spinach leaves in the bottom, followed by slices of tomato and mushroom.

Mix the egg white with a little salt and pepper and pour into the cracks. Cover with the grated cheese and bake in the oven for 30 minutes.

Gently place the egg yolk on top and bake for another 2 minutes.

Cut into quarters to serve.

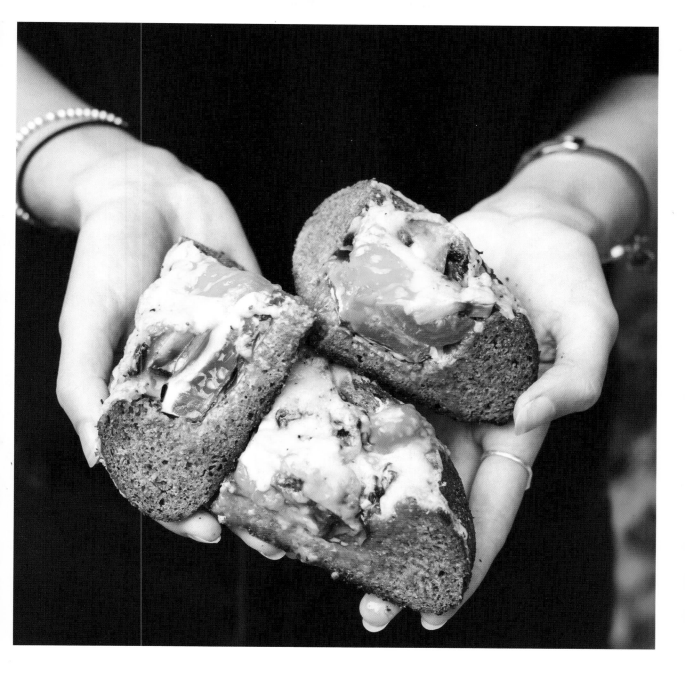

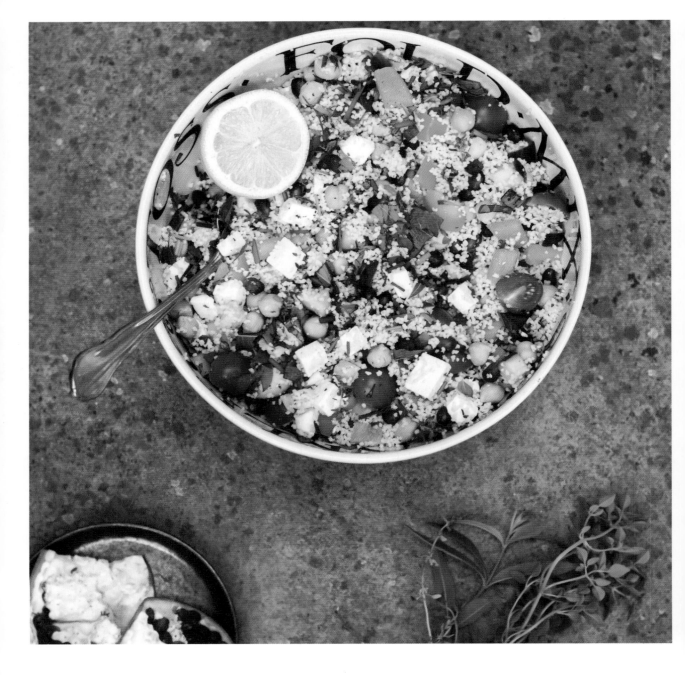

COUSCOUS SALAD

SERVES 6-8

- 200g couscous
- ½ vegetable stock cube
- ½ lemon, zested and juiced
- 2 tbsp olive oil
- 200g feta, cubed
- 150g cucumber, cubed
- 1 orange or yellow pepper, cubed
- 150g tomatoes, diced
- 1 x 400g tin of chickpeas, drained and rinsed
- 100g pomegranate seeds
- Large handful of fresh herbs (as many of the following as possible: basil, flat-leaf parsley, chives, oregano, mint, thyme, sage), finely sliced
- Salt and pepper
- Halved lemons, to serve

You don't see many wellness bloggers eating couscous . . . Maybe because it's not gluten-free? Couscous is made from wheat, so lots of gluten there. But it's one of the easiest and quickest grains to cook – just add hot water. Literally.

Measure out the couscous into a large bowl.

Mix 300ml of boiling water with the vegetable stock cube, the lemon zest and juice and the olive oil. Pour over the couscous and leave for 10 minutes.

Fluff up the couscous with a fork.

Add the feta, cucumber, pepper, tomatoes, chickpeas, pomegranate seeds and herbs to the couscous and season with salt and pepper. Stir to combine and serve with halved lemons.

 TIP Add a little hot stock to leftovers the next day to freshen them up.

HAZELNUT & CRANBERRY GRANOLA

SERVES 4-6

- 150g rolled oats (other kinds work well too)
- 30g ground flaxseed
- 50g chopped hazelnuts
- 50g whole hazelnuts
- 3 tbsp olive oil
- 4 tbsp maple syrup or rice syrup (maple is sweeter)
- 100g dried cranberries
- Yoghurt and fresh fruit, to serve

Oats are one of the few grains that pretty much everyone in wellness, from fitness bloggers to fake nutritionists, can agree are good for you. We've had overnight oats, zoats (porridge with shredded courgette) and proats (porridge with added protein). We've had an avalanche of porridge recipes, so I don't feel a particularly strong urge to contribute to that - pretty much anyone can make porridge. So here's some granola instead.

Preheat the oven to 150°C fan/170°C conventional/gas mark 3. Mix together the oats, flaxseed and chopped and whole hazelnuts.

Add the olive oil and syrup and mix into the dry ingredients until thoroughly combined.

Spread the mixture out quite thinly over a baking tray and bake in the oven for 15 minutes. The mixture should be crunchy by this point. If not, bake for another 5-10 minutes.

Add the cranberries and stir gently. Bake for another 5 minutes.

Allow to cool slightly before handling the mixture so that the clusters hold their shape.

Store in an airtight container and serve with yoghurt and fresh fruit for breakfast.

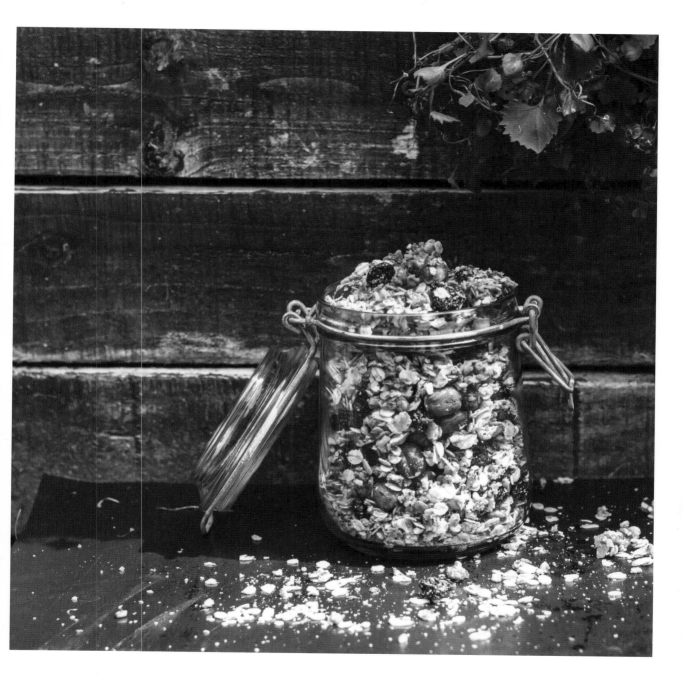

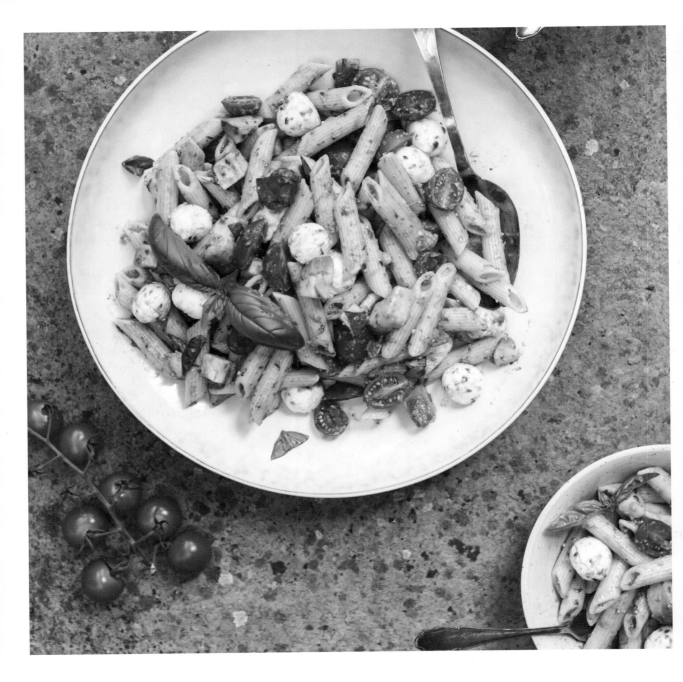

TRICOLORE PESTO PENNE

SERVES 4

- 250g penne (around 600g cooked)
- 95g basil pesto
- 150g plum tomatoes, halved
- 1 large avocado, cubed
- 150g mini mozzarella balls
- 1 tbsp fresh basil leaves, shredded

Pasta is an ideal, quick, no-fuss lunch or dinner option and this recipe is particularly speedy. I'm not even expecting you to make your own pesto, although you can if you want to, of course. Use regular, whole wheat or gluten-free pasta, I won't judge. Just make sure to cook it for 1 minute less than packet instructions to get perfectly al dente pasta that isn't overcooked!

Bring a large saucepan of salted water to the boil.

Add the penne and cook for 10 minutes (or 1 minute less than the packet states).

When cooked, drain the water from the penne and coat in pesto.

Add the tomatoes, avocado cubes, mozzarella balls and shredded basil leaves and mix together.

Serve immediately.

 TIP This recipe tastes great cold too! Simply refresh leftovers with a little extra pesto or olive oil.

SANDWICHES THREE WAYS

Cheesy sandwich
- ½ medium avocado, mashed
- Salt and pepper
- 3 slices of mature cheddar cheese
- ¼ red pepper
- Small handful of salad leaves

Yoghurty aubergine sandwich
- ½ small aubergine, sliced into rings
- Olive oil
- Salt and pepper
- 80g yoghurt
- 1 tsp chives
- 4-6 slices of cucumber
Sprinkling of cress

Smoked Tofu and Hummus Sandwich
- 40g hummus
- 50g firm smoked tofu, sliced
- 1 small carrot, grated
- Small handful of spinach leaves

In wellness, avocado toast is acceptable, but top with another slice of bread and it becomes something evil: a sandwich! Sandwiches are far too mainstream for wellness, but there's nothing to be afraid of. A sandwich can be a wonderful, nutritious meal. Here are three delocious examples of fillings to put between two slices of bread.

Cheesy sandwich

Season the avocado and spread three-quarters on one slice of bread and the rest on a second slice. Place the cheese slices on top of the thicker avocado, followed by the pepper and salad leaves, then put the second piece of bread on top.

Yoghurty aubergine sandwich

Drizzle the aubergine with olive oil and season. Heat a griddle pan until hot and grill the aubergine slices on both sides until cooked. Mix together the yoghurt and chives and season with salt and pepper Spread the yoghurt on two slices of bread. Place the aubergine on one of the pieces of bread, followed by the sliced cucumber and a sprinkling of cress, then put the second piece of bread on top.

Smoked tofu & hummus sandwich

Spread the hummus on two slices of bread. Place the tofu on one of the slices, followed by the carrot and spinach, then top with the second piece of bread.

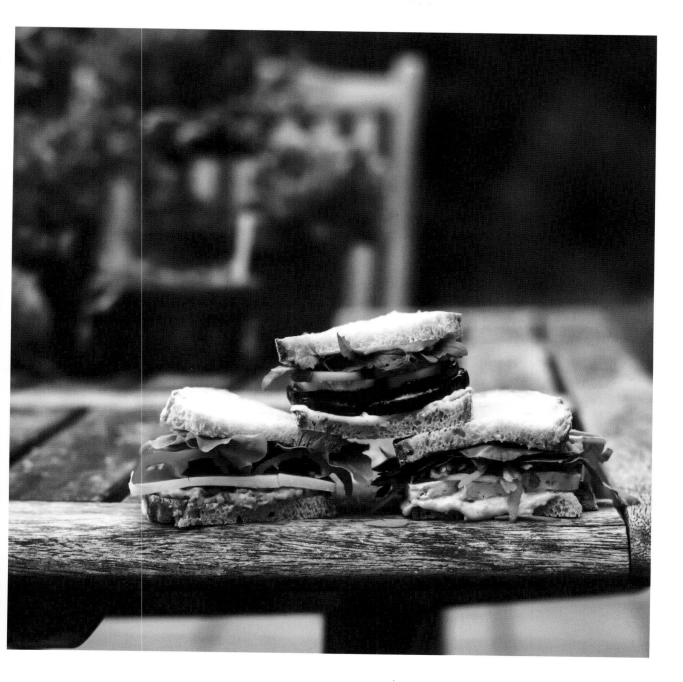

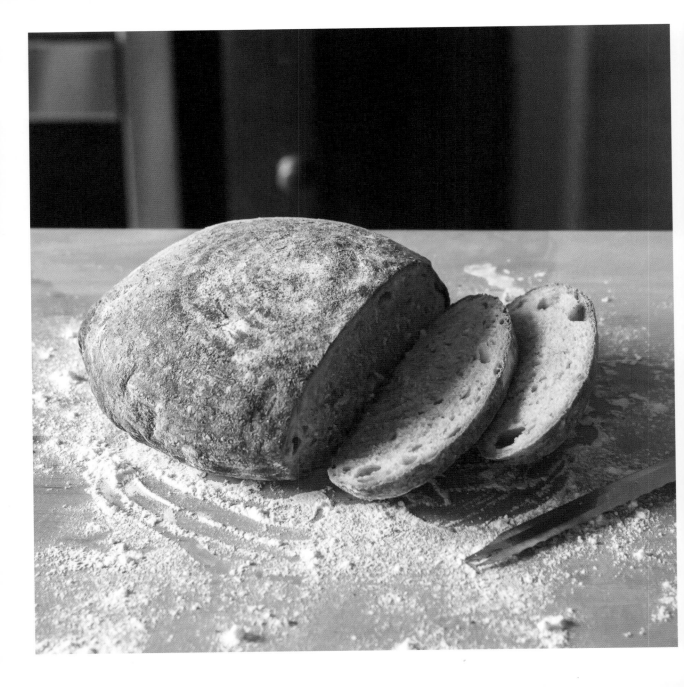

PIXIE'S BEGINNERS SOURDOUGH

MAKES 1 LOAF

For the leaven
- 20g starter
- 220g strong white flour

For the loaf
- 350g leaven
- 100g wholemeal bread flour
- 220g strong white flour
- 9g salt

You will need:
- A scraper
- A proving basket or large bowl
- A Dutch oven or two baking trays
- A lot of patience - this recipe takes 2 days to make!

I LOVE BREAD and I find making it very therapeutic. I learnt to make sourdough at the E5 Bakehouse in London, and that's where I get my starter every time I kill one (which happens more often than I care to admit). If you're a newbie to sourdough, start with a recipe like this, which focuses on white flour as it's much easier to bake with.

To make the leaven, mix together the starter and 170ml of lukewarm water, then add the flour and mix with your hands to combine. It should look like image 1. Cover the bowl with a tea towel and set aside for 8–24 hours, depending on the conditions; 8 hours if it's a warm sunny day or closer to 24 hours if it's a cold winter's day. You want it to be stringy and full of holes when you break the surface.

To make the loaf, weigh out 350g of the leaven you made the day before and add 210ml of water. Use your fingers to rub the mixture to combine it with the water until there are no lumps (see image 2). Don't use a rigorous stirring method; be gentle with it.

Add the wholemeal and white flours and combine into a single mass. Don't worry if it's still very sticky at this point (see image 3). Leave for 20 minutes.

Place the mixture on a floured surface, form a well and add the salt. Fold the edges of the dough over so the salt is inside and work the dough to disperse the salt. Place back in the bowl and leave for 30 minutes. It should now be a ball like in image 4. >

PIXIE'S BEGINNERS SOURDOUGH cont.

Stretch and fold a section of the dough (see images 5 and 6) without letting the dough break. This forms a rough triangle with the piece you've folded (the top of the triangle is in the centre of the dough and the two corners the edges); take hold of one of those corners and repeat the stretch and fold. Repeat this once all the way around. Flip the dough over and place your hands on either side of the dough. Move both hands in a clockwise motion, while tucking the dough slightly under, to form a ball shape (without it losing contact with the work surface). Place it back into the bowl and leave for 30 minutes.

Repeat the stretch and fold, leave for 30 minutes. Repeat the stretch and fold again, leave for 30 minutes. Form the dough into a ball and sprinkle generously with flour. Place it seam-side up in a proving basket (or a bowl with enough space for it to grow) (see image 7) and leave to prove for 60-90 minutes.

Preheat the oven to its highest temperature. Put a Dutch oven or lined baking tray in the oven to warm, then fill another baking tray with boiling water and place this in the bottom of the oven.

Carefully place the loaf in the hot Dutch oven or on the hot baking tray and bake for 30 minutes with the lid on the Dutch oven or with the tray of water, then for another 10 minutes without the lid or tray.

The loaf is ready when nicely browned on top (see image 8) and when the base sounds hollow when tapped. Leave to cool before slicing (see image 9).

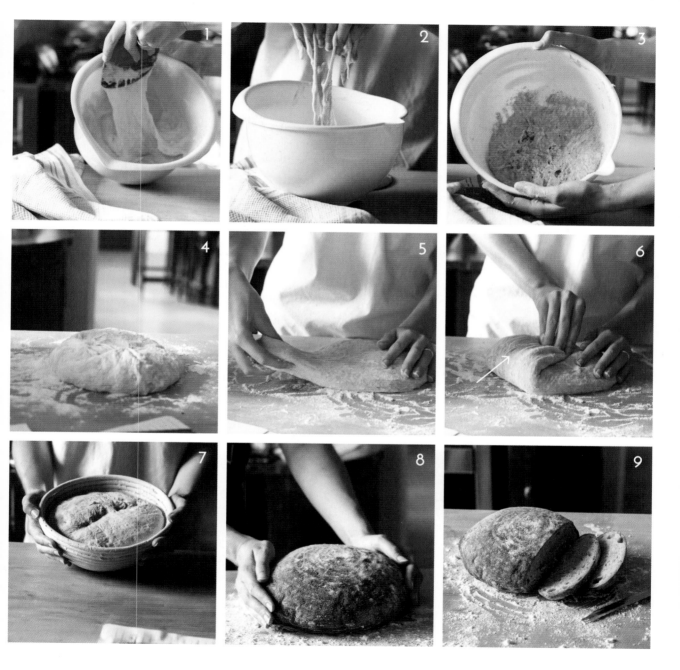

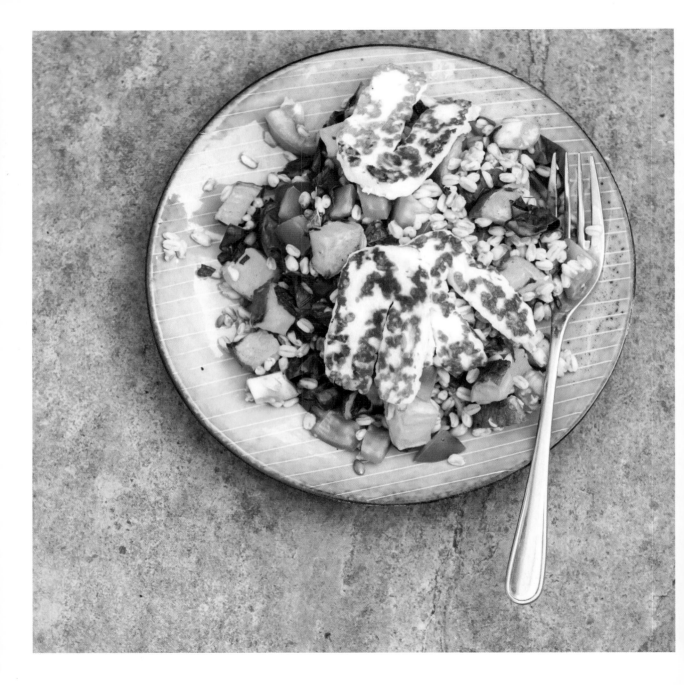

SPELT WITH HALLOUMI & SWEET POTATO

SERVES 2

- 200g sweet potatoes
- Olive oil
- Salt and pepper
- 150g pearled spelt
- 1 tbsp tahini
- 60g spinach leaves, roughly chopped
- 150g tomatoes, roughly chopped
- 1 tbsp fresh mint leaves, roughly chopped
- 100g halloumi

Spelt is a more unusual grain. Yes, it contains gluten, which is probably at least partly why it hasn't reached the same popularity level as quinoa. If you can't find spelt, rice would work very well instead.

Preheat the oven to 200°C fan/220°C conventional/gas mark 7.

Peel and chop the sweet potatoes into cubes and place on a lined baking tray. Drizzle with olive oil, season with salt and pepper and roast in the oven for 20–30 minutes, until soft.

Cook the spelt in a saucepan of boiling salted water for 20 minutes.

Drain any excess water and stir in the tahini, along with a little salt to taste.

Add the chopped spinach to the spelt. Replace the lid to let it wilt slightly.

Add the cooked sweet potato, tomatoes and chopped mint to the pan and mix everything together. Transfer to a serving dish or two plates.

Fry the halloumi in a dry frying pan and place on top of the salad. Serve immediately before the cheese becomes rubbery.

TIP If you are making this in advance, don't fry the halloumi until you're ready to eat.

TOMATO & COURGETTE RISOTTO

SERVES 4-6

- Olive oil
- 1 onion (around 110g), peeled and diced
- 1 vegetable stock cube
- 400g risotto rice
- 1 x 400g tin of chopped tomatoes
- 1 courgette (around 250g), coarsely grated
- 100g cherry tomatoes, halved
- 2 garlic cloves, peeled
- Large handful of fresh basil leaves
- Coarse sea salt
- 25g butter or vegan margarine
- 100g finely grated Parmesan, plus extra for sprinkling (leave out to make it vegan)

Most vegetarians will have had at least one bad risotto experience in their life. Mushroom risotto is the typical veggie option on a meat-focused menu, and it often feels like a cop-out. A risotto like this one was made for me at an event with chef Theo Randall, and it was the first time I tasted risotto and loved it. It was perfection. So, naturally, I went home and tried my best to recreate it from the vague instructions I remembered. I'd say it's just as good as his, but don't tell him that. Oh, and it's gluten-free!

Heat 2 tablespoons of olive oil in a wide, straight-sided frying pan over a medium heat. Cook the onion for around 5 minutes, making sure it doesn't burn.

In the meantime, cover the vegetable stock cube with 500ml of boiling water and stir until dissolved.

Add the rice to the frying pan and heat through, stirring continuously for a few minutes.

Add half the stock, stir thoroughly, then add the chopped tomatoes. Cook the rice for 15 minutes or 2 minutes less than recommended by the packet instructions, stirring continuously.

Cook the courgette separately in a little olive oil to remove any excess moisture. >

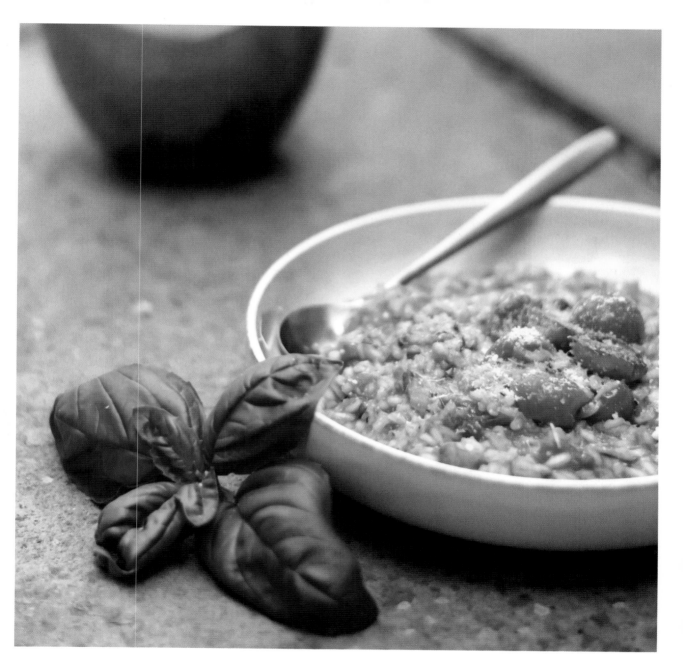

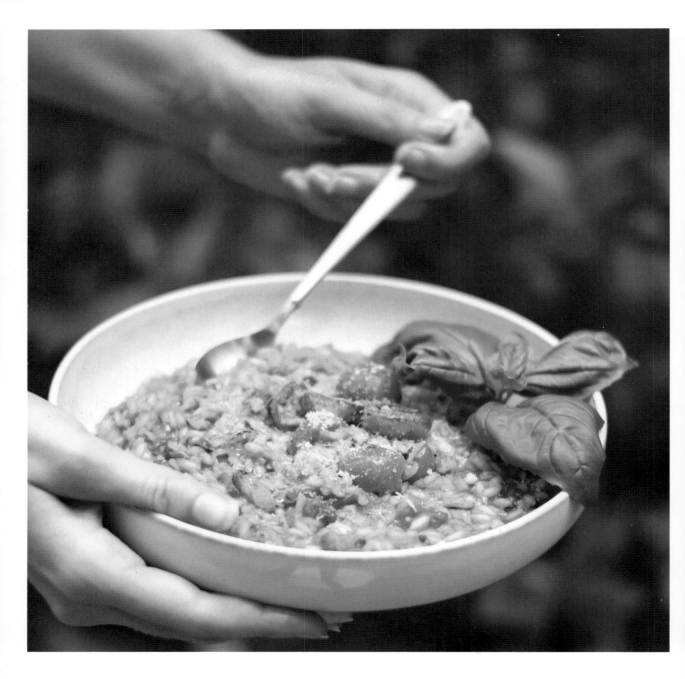

TOMATO & COURGETTE RISOTTO cont.

It's a bit of a juggling act, but stir both pans continuously to avoid the rice sticking to the bottom of the pan (turn down the heat if necessary) and to avoid burning the courgette. If the rice gets too dry, add a some of the remaining stock, a little at a time. If it bubbles too much, turn down the heat a little.

Once the courgette has lost most of its moisture, stir it into the rice. Add a little more oil to the pan that the courgettes were in and gently cook the cherry tomatoes until soft.

In a pestle and mortar, crush the garlic and basil to a paste with a little sea salt and add to the risotto. If you don't have a pestle and mortar, then use a small food processor or finely chopping by hand would work too.

When the rice has been cooking for 15 minutes, taste the risotto. It should be al dente, not completely soft. If it's ready, turn off the heat and stir in the cherry tomatoes. Stir through the butter and half the Parmesan, if using.

Serve immediately, adding a sprinkling of Parmesan and a final drizzle of olive oil (trust me on this one, don't skip it) to each individual plate.

VANILLA WAFFLES WITH STRAWBERRY COMPOTE

MAKES 1 WAFFLE

- 100g chopped strawberries (fresh or frozen)
- 1 tbsp maple syrup
- 50g plain or wholemeal flour
- 1 tsp baking powder
- Pinch of salt
- 1 tsp vanilla bean paste or essence
- 1 tbsp sugar or 1 tsp stevia
- 1 egg, beaten
- 50ml milk (cows, oat or almond)
- Greek yoghurt (optional)

I used to make vegan and gluten-free pancakes, and now I look back and have no idea how I managed that. Pancakes and waffles taste so much better with gluten in them. If you don't have a waffle iron, you can easily make these into pancakes instead!

Put the strawberries and maple syrup into a small saucepan, along with a splash of water if using fresh berries. Cook gently until it becomes thick and jam-like. This will take anywhere between 5–20 minutes depending on the berries.

Mix together the rest of the ingredients (minus the yoghurt) and stir until thoroughly combined.

Pour into a preheated waffle iron and cook for around 5 minutes, until golden brown.

When ready, serve with the strawberry compote and yoghurt (if using).

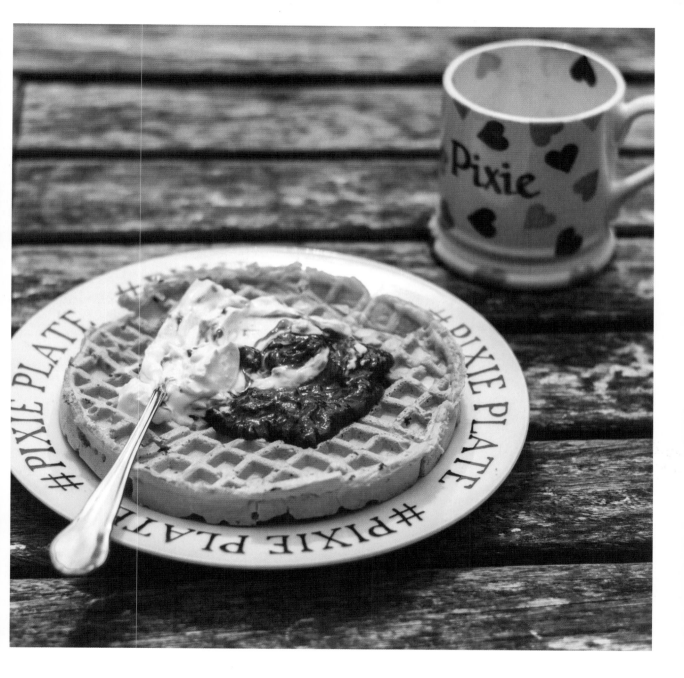

Detox

THE DETOXING MYTH

How many times have you seen the 'January detox' claims so far this year? Or 'spring detox' or 'detox to get that summer body' or even 'detox your weekend away'?

Whether it's juice cleanses, detox teas, coffee enemas or intense doses of intravenous vitamins, the 'detox' trend is pervasive. It has especially thrived on social media, with some companies having tens of thousands of followers and seemingly endless funds for celebrity endorsements.

These 'detox' methods all claim to be able to rid your body of toxins in some way. Let's examine these methods one by one and see what they have to offer. . .

JUICE CLEANSES

The principle with juice cleanses is pretty straightforward: no food for several days, just drink juice. But not just any old juice, oh no, it has to be raw, organic, cold-pressed juice because God forbid you should drink some cheap supermarket own-brand orange juice.

I looked at some of the top search results for juice cleanses and took some direct quotes as to what these cleanses claim to be able to offer you; it's quite impressive. These cleanses claim to be able to 'boost your detoxification systems' (but don't say how), 'flush out toxins' (which ones though?), 'hydrate your cells' (like how water does?), make your skin 'glow', help you lose weight and gain energy. They also claim to give your digestive system a break, demonstrating a clear misunderstanding of how the human body works. Seriously, that's not how it works.

Some websites make more specific claims, like being able to 'detox your body' from heavy metals. Let's touch on heavy metals. You need some of these heavy metals, like zinc, copper and manganese, in small amounts to survive. But too much is dangerous. Heavy metal poisoning has very specific symptoms, which vary with the type of metal, so lumping symptoms of 'heavy metal poisoning' together is a sure sign of nutribollocks. If you have a form of heavy metal poisoning you need a trip to A&E; a green juice isn't going to help you there.

These claims, unsurprisingly, are all vague and unverified. Sure, you're getting lots of nutrients in, but you could just as easily get all of those from food. A juice diet is lacking in fibre, can be high in free sugars if heavily fruit juice-based (don't forget, according to the SACN guidelines fruit juices count as free sugars) and is likely to be low in protein. None of this is a real problem over the course of a day or a couple of days, except that the lack of sodium can make you feel dizzy, and if you're having just pure vegetable juices there's a complete lack of carbs, so you can feel really tired – the opposite of what they're promising.

Juice cleanses are expensive (oh hey, another example of the elitism of the wellness industry) and don't create positive long-term lifestyle habits. Even if you're not using them to 'detox' but just to lose some weight, chances are you'll just gain the weight back again once you go back to eating food instead of juicing.

DETOX TEAS

At risk of losing my impartiality (not sure I had that much to begin with to be honest), I really hate detox teas. To me they are everything that is wrong with social media rolled into one giant ball of celebrity-endorsed dung. An appropriate metaphor, as you're about to find out.

If you've never come across detox teas before, I salute you, and please tell me where you've been hiding that you've managed to avoid this awful product. I want to go there.

Detox teas are herbal teas that are meant to be drunk 2–3 times a day, either around 30 minutes before each meal, or once in the morning and once at night.

Often these teas, or at least the evening brew, contain a herbal laxative called senna. The laxative means you lose water weight and extra stools, and can therefore trick you into thinking it's effective for weight loss. It's not. You are literally just losing water weight, and when you stop the laxative, you just put that water weight back on. Laxatives don't cause fat loss or 'detox' the body [1].

Not only that, but senna can cause multiple side-effects, some of which are even listed on 'teatox' websites. We're talking dehydration, fatigue, dizziness, colon damage, pain, cramps, diarrhoea and laxative-dependency [1]. The latter is of special concern as laxatives shouldn't be used for more than 2 weeks, and these detox teas are often sold in monthly or 28-day packages. So you might find that after your 'detox month' you're constipated, which is not a good position to be in.

Detox tea companies recommend following a calorie-controlled diet and exercising regularly alongside drinking their tea. So ask yourself, what's likely to actually be having an effect here?

ACTIVATED CHARCOAL

Activated charcoal is made from coconut shells, wood or peat heated to high temperatures and combined with gas or an activating agent. This 'activates' it as it increases the surface area through the creation of lots of tiny holes, which allows it to bind to various substances and prevents them from being absorbed into the bloodstream.

Activated charcoal is sometimes used to help treat poisoning or drug overdoses, so it's serious stuff! This also means it can interact with drugs you're taking such as painkillers, birth control or prescription medication, so be careful! [2]. Having said that, it won't prevent hangovers as it doesn't bind to alcohol, and alcohol is absorbed too quickly for charcoal to be able to have any effect [3].

Activated charcoal won't 'detox' or cleanse your blood as the charcoal particles are too large to be absorbed into the bloodstream; it goes straight into the gut and then out of you.

So what's the harm? Well, it may also reduce the absorbance of some nutrients from food, so you could be missing out on important vitamins and minerals if you have it at the same time as food – in a charcoal latte for example [4].

Overall, activated charcoal has some supporting evidence, but this is in life-threatening medical situations, not for when you're just feeling run down and 'full of toxins'.

EATING ORGANIC

I've often seen people claim we should eat organic to 'detox' from pesticide residues. Let's set something straight from the start: organic doesn't mean pesticide-free. In fact, there's a long list of pesticides, herbicides, etc. which are approved by the Soil Association in the UK. Organic doesn't tell you how much crops are sprayed or how often; it simply tells you about the type of pesticide used, namely natural ones rather than the artificial ones allowed in conventional farming practices.

Pesticides are toxic, yes. Of course they are, that's the whole point of them. The reason we use them is to kill unwanted living organisms. But just because they're highly toxic to insects doesn't necessarily mean the same applies to humans. Chocolate is toxic to dogs but you don't see people using that as an excuse for us not to eat it.

There is no relationship between the 'naturalness' of a pesticide and its toxicity to humans. Some natural pesticides are more toxic than artificial ones, and some are less. For example, organic farmers can use copper solutions to treat fungal diseases, and this copper stays toxic in the soil, unlike more modern biodegradable pesticides.

Synthetic pesticides are rigorously tested for safety and take years to come to market as a result. Non-organic produce isn't 'saturated with chemicals'; not only is that fearmongering and exaggerated, it also doesn't make sense as a business practice – pesticides cost money! The levels of pesticide residues that are found in our food are completely safe and easily managed by the body. This brilliant quote sums it up for me: 'We calculate that 99.99% (by weight) of the pesticides in the American diet are chemicals that plants produce to defend themselves'. [5] That's only 0.01% pesticides that we add, both natural and synthetic. Doesn't feel that significant now.

I will say it a hundred times until it sticks: just because something is natural doesn't mean it's inherently good or better for you than something that isn't natural. Your body doesn't recognise foods or food sources, it recognises chemical structures and chemical bonds.

Organic produce also isn't necessarily healthier or more nutrient-dense. Systematic reviews comparing organic vs conventional produce showed no evidence for differences in nutritional content [6][7]. Yes, you'll find individual studies that show organic has higher amounts of specific nutrients in specific crops, but these aren't necessarily representative of the bigger picture, and could simply be down to soil type, geographical location, seasonality or bad study design. Let's not forget that the organic industry sponsors research, and that should make us sceptical of those results.

Overall, the evidence says that organic food is not necessarily better for you or better tasting than conventional produce. Resorting to eating organic to 'detox' from pesticide residues isn't going to work unless you only choose produce that uses no pesticides at all. And even then, it doesn't really matter, as pesticide residues are found on foods at a level which is safe for us to consume and your body is extremely well-equipped to deal with these residues.

Just because
something
is natural
doesn't make it
inherently 'good'.

COFFEE ENEMAS

Do I have to explain this one? Essentially it involves brewing some organic coffee and using 'chemical-free' filtered water (do they realise coffee is made up of over 100 different chemicals?), letting it cool, pouring it into an enema bag, then lying on the floor with a connecting tube up your rectum. You let gravity do its work for around 15 minutes. This is claimed to 'reduce toxicity', 'cleanse and heal the colon', 'help with depression' and 'increase energy levels'.

Ironically, despite claims to 'heal' the colon, a coffee enema might actually do the opposite. Along with a risk of rectal perforation, side effects include infections, severe electrolyte imbalances, colitis, brain abscess, heart failure and internal burning. People have died as a result of coffee enemas from some of these side effects. What a way to go.

Any 'sludge' (eww) that comes out is basically diarrhoea. I mean, why would you voluntarily give yourself diarrhoea?! That's not toxins, that's just shit. Literally. You don't need to detox your digestive system; if the organs aren't working right, you'll know thanks to symptoms like jaundice or blood in your stool. Coffee won't help.

Why it's recommended to have coffee as an enema rather than simply drinking it is beyond me. There's no reason to suspect you'd react differently to coffee orally or up your rectum. Once the caffeine has been absorbed, how are your cells supposed to know where it went in? They don't. Obviously.

Perhaps the worst part about this procedure is that it's used in Gerson therapy to 'cure' cancer by 'detoxing' you. I am not a religious person, but I strongly believe there's a special circle of hell reserved for the peddlers of fake cancer treatments. Coffee definitely doesn't cure cancer.

IV VITAMIN INFUSIONS

This is a much more recent phenomenon made popular by cash-rich, time-poor celebrities getting their latest health fix. Vitamin concoctions are made up according to your needs (or select a prepared formula) and injected straight into your bloodstream over the course of about an hour.

These infusions are claimed to help with stress and jetlag, boost energy levels and stimulate the immune system.

There are no clinical studies that show IV vitamin infusions have meaningful effects beyond simple placebo. We can get them all from a balanced diet, plus excess vitamins are just excreted in the urine. We are designed, so to speak, to absorb vitamins through our digestive system, not into our veins.

Risks from these procedures include bruising, infection and vein inflammation, and wrong doses can lead to sudden cardiac death. Very high doses of vitamins (hypervitaminosis) can actually be just as harmful as vitamin deficiencies, with severe cases requiring hospitalisation.

LEMON WATER

We're supposed to absorb vitamins through our digestive system.

Having a glass of warm water with lemon is recommended by a whole host of Instagram bloggers and wellness warriors, but why? Often, it's simply claimed to be 'good for you' without any validation, but I've also seen more specific claims such as 'flushing out toxins'.

Lemon water is claimed to 'wake up your liver' first thing in the morning. Your liver doesn't need waking up. If your liver went to sleep every time you did, you probably wouldn't wake up again. Your liver is always awake!

Lemon water is also claimed to be 'alkalising', which makes no sense considering it contains a fair dose of citric acid, which has led to dentists warning against the practice on a daily basis as the acid can wear away tooth enamel and damage your teeth. The claims about 'alkalising', though, are a whole other story for a whole other chapter . . .

Detoxification is a scientific principle that's been hijacked by the wellness industry, and is wrapped in a scientific banner in an attempt to give the treatments and practitioners credibility

YOUR BODY'S NATURAL DETOXIFICATION SYSTEM

Metabolic processes in your body can produce harmful substances, which can be made less toxic through a variety of reactions. This is your body's natural detoxification system. There are a group of around thirty detoxification enzymes in your body, of which important ones include P450 oxidases, glucuronosyltransferases (try pronouncing that one, I can barely spell it!) and glutathione-S-transferases.

There are three phases of detoxification:

Phase 1 – modification, usually oxidation reactions (adding oxygen or losing electrons) and most commonly performed by P450 enzymes.

Phase 2 – conjugation, basically joining two things together, which usually involves making something more water-soluble so it can be more easily transported in the blood and removed via the kidneys.

Phase 3 – excretion, usually via the kidneys then the urine.

The liver does most of the work here, but the kidneys, lungs and skin also help, particularly with more localised toxicity. Every biological tissue has some detoxification ability. This system works night and day, 24/7, non-stop. A juice cleanse or special tea doesn't help it along; if it didn't work properly you'd end up with symptoms so severe you'd be hospitalised and could end up dead.

IT'S ALL NUTRIBOLLOCKS

Notice what's missing from all of the 'detox' methods mentioned? A mechanism maybe? I'd even be content with them naming toxins, but even that seems to be beyond people.

All you need to 'detox' are a liver and kidneys, which work 24/7 to make sure you don't die.

You just need a liver and kidneys to detox, they do all the work, performing complex reactions to convert toxic substances into ones that are safe for excretion. Most 'detox' products don't even mention which toxins they're getting rid of as they don't get rid of any. Why do people claim detoxes worked for them? Aside from being paid to say so on social media, of course. It could be that they've been eating a healthier diet, a placebo effect or simply a natural recovery from symptoms which would have occurred regardless. Going on a detox often provides a placebo effect which makes people believe they are healthier – they might be if they're making positive changes to their diets – but that's not due to a special tea or enema!

On the flip side, any negative symptoms that are often associated with things like juice cleanses are always twisted into simply being signs that the detox is working. Whilst this is a clever marketing tactic, it's also absolutely rubbish. If you're feeling dizzy and nauseous, you're not 'detoxing', you're probably just really hungry and need food.

Detoxification is a scientific principle that's been hijacked by the wellness industry, and is wrapped in a scientific banner in an attempt to give the treatments and practitioners credibility. On websites advertising juice cleanses or coffee enemas, you'll see references to specific enzymes and organs and pathways, but put together in a way that doesn't actually happen or isn't even possible. It's a great attempt to sound scientific, and sadly is often successful

The bottom line is: if you like green juice then enjoy it as part of a balanced diet, drink herbal teas because you like the taste, eat organic if you prefer the taste or enjoy the community aspect, take a multivitamin (orally please) or see a medical professional if you're worried about your vitamin levels, and please for the love of all living things, pour your coffee down your throat, not up your rectum.

So, is there anything you can do to help your liver with its detoxification pathways? Yes. Strangely, the best way to help your body deal better with toxins is to make sure you ingest some. Alcohol is technically a toxin. But population studies have shown that people who drink moderately and in small amounts have a longer life expectancy than teetotallers and those who drink excessively [8]. While it's probably unethical for me to encourage alcohol consumption, I'm not going to say you have to give it up either. This effect of alcohol on life expectancy is likely to be partly related to the social aspect of drinking, but also due to the fact that alcohol is a poison.

Let me explain. In the same way that being around cats and dogs and playing outside in the dirt at a young age is beneficial for the immune system because it increases the variety of bacteria you're exposed to, consuming a tiny bit of poison like alcohol primes the enzymes in your liver to deal better with any other poisons.

But if alcohol isn't your thing, then how about broccoli? Brassicas (of which broccoli is a member) contain an inactive form of cyanide, which becomes activated on digestion. Eating broccoli provides a tiny amount of poison, which primes the liver's enzymes. Broccoli is one of many foods that can have this kind of effect, and on the following pages I'll share some recipes which contain foods and plant chemicals that can prime your liver's enzymes, whilst also making you feel good. These aren't 'detoxifying' foods, these are simply foods that may have more of an effect on your liver than other foods due to their chemical make-up. The best thing you can do to support your liver is simply eat a balanced diet and not go too crazy on the alcohol.

The best thing you can do to support your liver is eat a balanced diet.

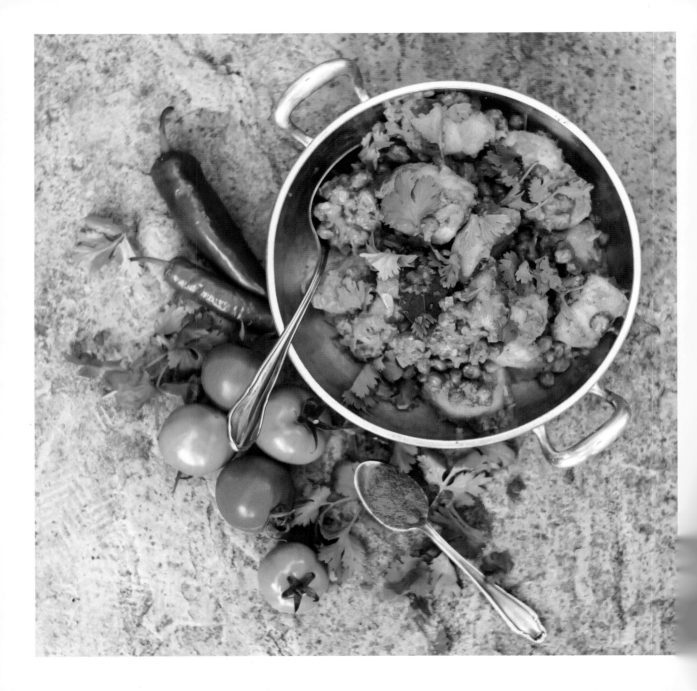

ALOO DUM

SERVES 4

- 800g potatoes (around 700g once peeled)
- 40g butter or 2 tbsp coconut oil
- 1 onion (around 110g), peeled and finely diced
- 1 bay leaf
- 4 garlic cloves, peeled and crushed
- 1 tbsp ground or minced ginger
- 2 tsp ground turmeric
- 1 tsp ground cumin
- 1 tsp ground coriander
- Pinch of chilli powder
- 200g passata
- 150g frozen peas
- 1 tsp garam masala
- Salt
- Fresh coriander leaves, to serve

The onions and garlic in this recipe contain sulphur, which is required for the phase-2 detoxification pathway in the liver. So while this recipe won't 'detox' you, it does provide key nutrients your body needs to make detoxification enzymes. There are also a whole load of delicious spices here, but don't worry if you don't have them all, just try to include as many of them as possible.

Peel the potatoes and cut them into large cubes (around 3cm). Bring a medium deep saucepan of salted water to the boil and boil the potatoes for 10 minutes.

Melt half the butter or coconut oil in a large shallow saucepan over a medium heat. Add the onion and bay leaf and cook for 5 minutes. Add the garlic and ginger and cook for 5 minutes, stirring.

Drain the potatoes and add them back to the deep pan. Add the remaining butter or coconut oil along with a teaspoon of turmeric and return the pan to the heat. Fry for 5 minutes.

Add the rest of the spices (cumin, coriander, chilli and the rest of the turmeric) to the shallow pan with the onions and stir for 1 minute. Add the passata and the potatoes to the shallow pan, cover with a lid and gently cook for 10 minutes.

Stir in the frozen peas to thaw them and the garam masala. Season with salt and finish with fresh coriander.

BLACK DAHL

SERVES 3-4

- 250g black beluga lentils
- 25g butter or coconut oil
- 1 small onion (around 100g), peeled and finely diced
- 1 bay leaf
- 2 cardamom pods (don't worry if you don't have these)
- 2 garlic cloves
- 1 tbsp ground or minced ginger
- 1 tsp ground coriander
- 1 tsp ground cumin
- 1 tsp chilli powder
- 50g tomato purée
- 1 vegetable stock cube
- Salt
- 1-2 tsp garam masala
- 200ml double cream (or use oat cream)
- Butter, to serve (optional)

If you've ever been to Dishoom in London you'll understand the wonder that is black dahl. I don't have the time or inclination to cook something for 24 hours, so although my version isn't quite as good, I think it comes reasonably close. Onions and garlic are also a source of sulphur, which your liver needs for its detoxification enzymes.

Rinse the lentils until the water runs clear.

Melt the butter or coconut oil in a medium-sized saucepan and cook the diced onion for 5 minutes, along with the bay leaf and cardamom pods (if using).

Peel and crush the garlic and add to the pan along with the ginger. Cook for another 5 minutes.

Add the coriander, cumin and chilli powder and stir for a minute. Add the tomato purée and stir until thoroughly combined.

Add the stock cube, lentils and around 500ml of water. Bring to a gentle simmer, and cook for at least 30 minutes, ideally around 2 hours, adding more water regularly as needed.

Season well with salt and garam masala. Add the cream, and some extra butter if you feel like making it extra creamy! Stir until well combined and serve.

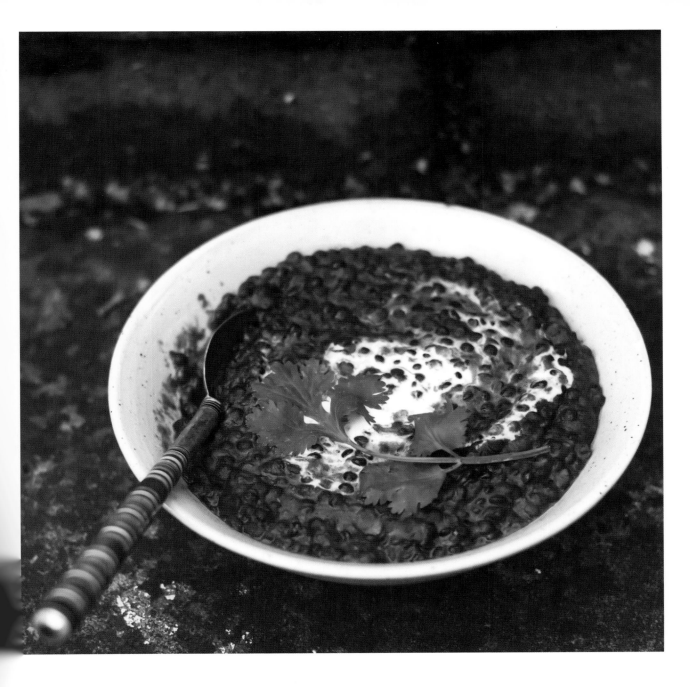

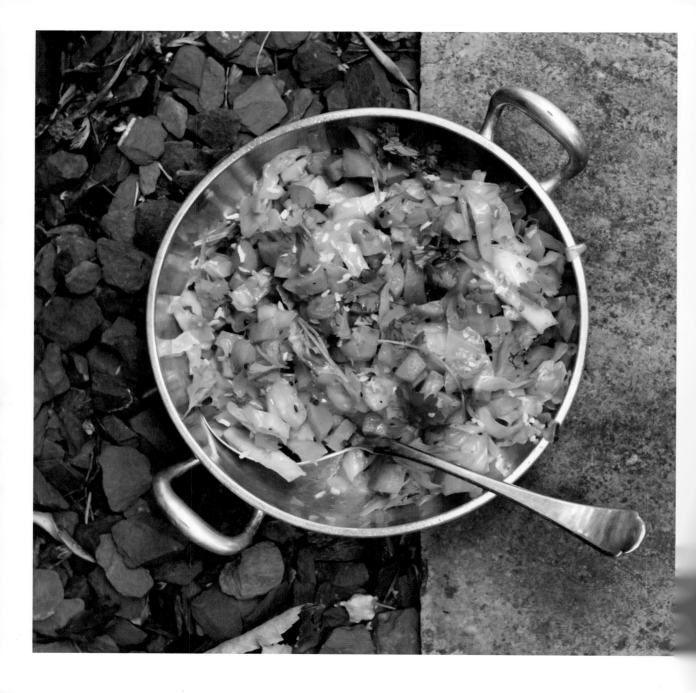

CABBAGE & CARROT CURRY

SERVES 3-4

- 2 carrots (around 240g)
- 250g white cabbage
- 2 tbsp coconut oil
- 1 tsp cumin seeds
- 1 tbsp ground ginger
- 1 tsp ground turmeric
- 1 tsp salt
- 1 fresh green chilli
- 1 tbsp desiccated or fresh coconut (optional)

This is the quickest curry recipe I've ever come up with. From start to finish, it takes about fifteen minutes, so it's great for when you're short on time. If you're one of those people who can handle curry on a hangover, this recipe is a great one, as cabbage is a member of the brassica family, and as such contains glucosinolates and other phytochemicals which encourage your liver's detoxification enzymes.

Dice the carrot finely (less than 1cm cubes) and finely slice the cabbage.

Heat the oil and cumin seeds in a wide-bottomed saucepan.

When the seeds are sizzling, add the rest of the spices and stir for 30 seconds.

Add the cabbage and carrot, and cook gently with the lid on for 5–7 minutes, until slightly tender but still crunchy.

Slice the chilli and stir in for another minute.

Add the coconut (if using) and serve.

CRUCIFEROUS TACOS WITH AVOCADO-YOGHURT DRESSING

MAKES 8 TACOS

- 2 tsp paprika
- 2 tsp ground cumin
- ½ tsp salt
- 1 tsp garlic powder or granules
- ½ tsp chilli powder or flakes (optional)
- 2 tbsp lime juice
- 3 tbsp olive oil
- 250g broccoli
- 250g cauliflower
- 1 x 400g tin of chickpeas, drained and rinsed
- 8 taco shells

For the dressing
- 1 medium avocado
- 200g natural yoghurt
- Juice of 1 lime
- Salt and pepper

Broccoli and cauliflower are both members of the brassica family, which contain phytochemicals such as glucosinolates. This chemical contains sulphur, which is required for the body's phase-2 detoxification pathways, and new research is currently underway to determine whether it has anti-cancer properties.

Preheat the oven to 200°C fan/220°C conventional/gas mark 6. Mix together the paprika, cumin, salt, garlic, chilli (if using), lime juice and olive oil to form a marinade.

Cut the broccoli and cauliflower into small florets. Spread over a baking tray with the chickpeas. Pour the marinade over the vegetables and toss to coat. Roast them in the oven for 30 minutes.

Meanwhile, make the avocado-yoghurt dressing. Place the avocado, yoghurt and lime juice in a food processor. (If you don't have one just mash with a fork until smooth.) Season with salt and pepper to taste. Place into a serving bowl.

Warm the taco shells for 30 seconds in a microwave. I'm a big fan of self-assembly when it comes to tacos, so I recommend placing everything in serving bowls in the middle of the table.

TIP Serve with chicken for extra protein.

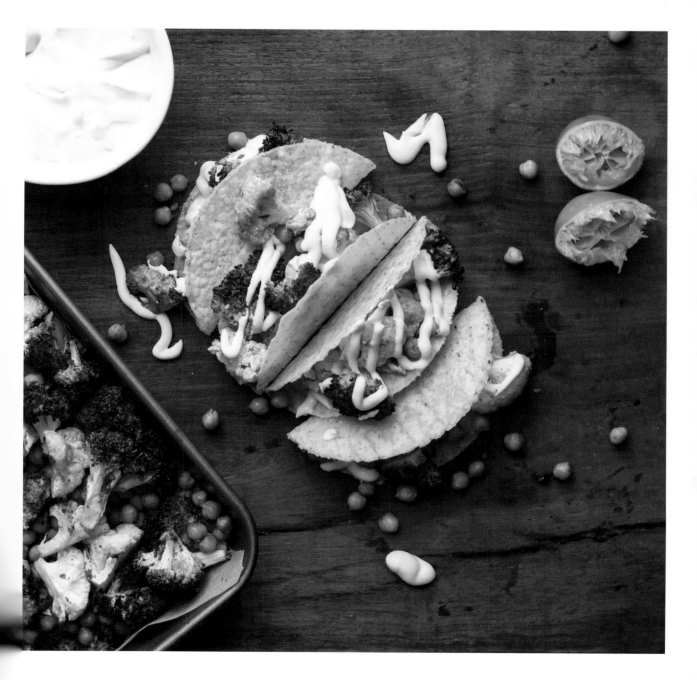

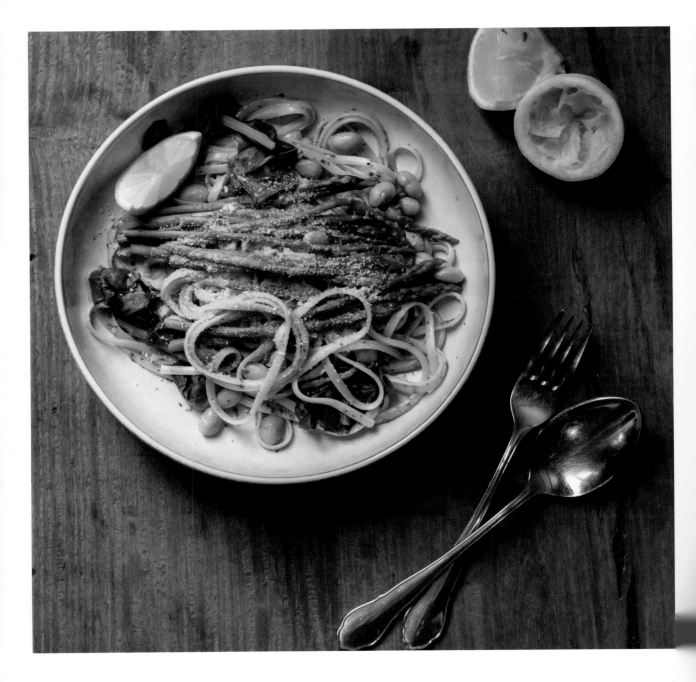

GREENS & LEMON LINGUINE

SERVES 2

- 150g linguine
- 1 garlic clove, peeled
- 20g fresh basil
- 2 tbsp olive oil
- ½ lemon, zested and juiced
- Salt and pepper
- 200g fine asparagus, woody stems removed (or 150g tips)
- 80g frozen edamame beans
- 30g spinach leaves
- Grated Parmesan or vegetarian hard cheese, to serve
- Lemon wedges, to serve

This recipe uses crushed garlic, which helps release the phytochemical allicin, an organosulphate (so it contains sulphur), which has been linked to a range of health benefits. As it contains sulphur, it also provides a building block for the detoxification enzymes in the liver. Not to mention it taste delicious when mixed with basil and lemon!

Bring one large and one small pot of salted water to the boil. Cook the linguine in the large pot for 7 minutes.

In a food processor, blend together the garlic, basil, olive oil and lemon zest and juice, with a pinch of salt and pepper. Taste and add more seasoning if needed.

Cook the asparagus and edamame in the small pot for 3–5 minutes.

With 2 minutes left, add the spinach to the vegetables to wilt slightly. Drain most of the water from the linguine, and add the lemony sauce. Toss to coat.

Drain the vegetables. Divide the linguine and vegetables between two bowls, and add a sprinkling of Parmesan, along with an extra drizzle of oil and sprinkling of salt if needed. Serve with lemon wedges.

TIP This would taste great with salmon added too.

MOROCCAN-STYLE BEAN STEW

SERVES 4

- Olive oil
- 1 onion (around 110g), peeled and finely diced
- 2 garlic cloves
- 1 tsp ground cinnamon
- 2 tsp ground cumin
- 2 tbsp ground coriander
- 2 tsp paprika
- ½ tsp chilli flakes
- 50g dates, stoned
- 200g carrots, cubed
- 250g sweet potato, peeled and cubed
- 1x 400g tin of chopped tomatoes
- 1 vegetable stock cube
- 1 orange or yellow pepper, chopped into 2cm cubes
- 1 x 400g tin of chickpeas, drained and rinsed
- 50g spinach leaves, chopped
- Salt and pepper
- Cooked rice, to serve
- Coriander leaves, to serve

It's all very well talking about the sulphur in onions and garlic and the way they help build the liver's detoxification enzymes, which they do, but enzymes are made of proteins and this recipe gives you all the amino acids your body needs by combining chickpeas with rice to form a complete protein source!

Heat a glug of oil in a large saucepan over a medium heat. Add the onion and cook for 5 minutes.

Peel and crush the garlic and add to the pan along with the spices. Stir for 1 minute. Add the dates, carrots and sweet potato and stir for 1 minute.

Add the chopped tomatoes along with a can full of water and the vegetable stock cube. Leave to simmer for 15–20 minutes, until the sweet potato and carrots are quite soft. If serving with rice, start cooking it at this point.

Add the chopped pepper and chickpeas to the pan and simmer for another 10 minutes.

Remove the pan from the heat and stir in the chopped spinach to wilt. Season to taste with salt and pepper.

Serve with rice and fresh coriander.

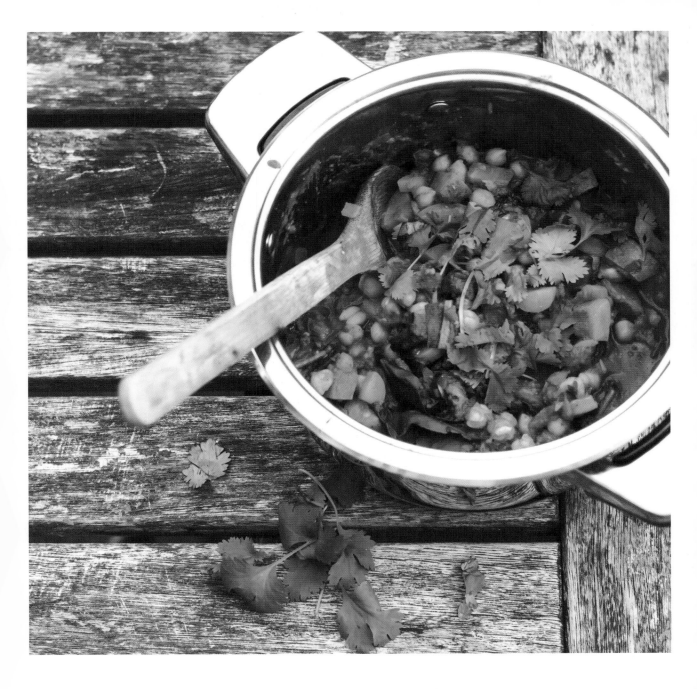

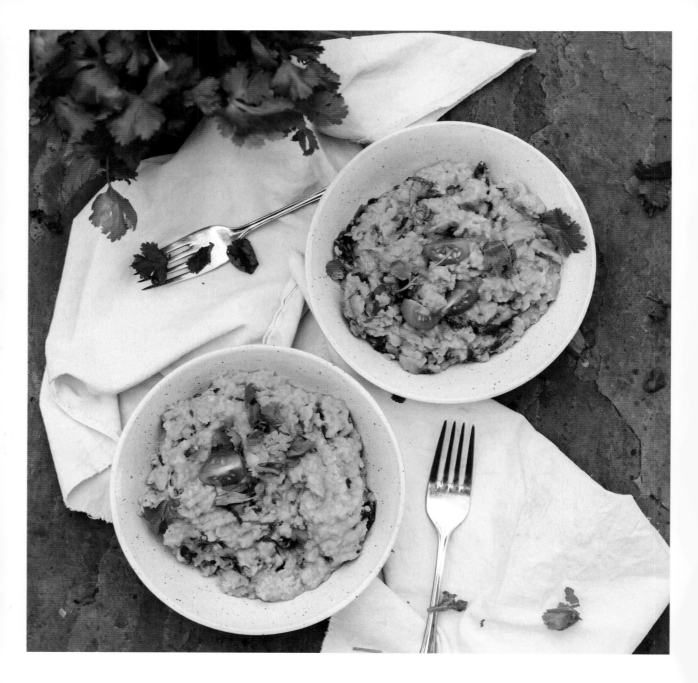

SPINACH & KALE DHAL

SERVES 4

- 400g red split lentils
- 1 tbsp coconut oil or ghee or vegetable oil
- 1 white onion (around 100g), peeled and diced
- 2 garlic cloves
- 1 tbsp ground ginger
- 1 tsp ground coriander
- ½ tsp chilli flakes
- 1 tbsp ground turmeric
- 1 tsp ground cumin
- ½ tsp ground cinnamon
- 1 vegetable stock cube
- 1 tomato (around 150g), diced
- 100g spinach leaves
- 50g roughly chopped kale
- Salt
- 1-2 tsp garam masala
- Fresh coriander leaves, to serve

I love dhal. I fell in love with it in India, of course, and have been obsessed with it ever since. I like using a combination of spinach and kale, because the spinach wilts until it's barely there, whereas the kale holds its shape a lot better, so the two complement each other nicely. Plus, there's the fact that kale is a member of the brassica family, and as much as it tastes vile raw, when cooked it's actually pretty decent.

Rinse the lentils until the water runs clear. Heat the oil or ghee in a medium saucepan over a medium heat.

Add the onion and reduce the heat to medium-low. Cook for 10 minutes. Peel and crush the garlic and add to the pan along with the ginger. Stir for a minute.

Add the rest of the spices (but not the garam masala) and stir for another minute. Dissolve the stock cube in 500ml of boiling water, then add to the pan along with the lentils.

Let it gently bubble away for 5 minutes, then add the diced tomato. After another 5 minutes, add the spinach and kale. Cook for another 5 minutes or so (around 15 minutes in total), until the lentils are cooked.

Turn off the heat and season with salt and garam masala. Taste and add more garam masala and salt if needed. Serve with fresh coriander.

MEDITERRANEAN STUFFED BUTTERNUT SQUASH

SERVES 4

- 1 butternut squash (around 1.2kg), halved and seeds removed
- Olive oil
- 100g quinoa (or 200g cooked grains)
- 1 lemon, halved
- 120g feta
- 80g sundried tomatoes
- 1 x 400g tin of chickpeas, drained and rinsed
- 30g spinach leaves
- Salt and pepper

Squash is a popular 'detox' food for some reason, along with lemons. I'm guessing the vitamin C probably has something to do with it, as vitamin C has an almost cult-like following. To be fair, vitamin C is important for liver function and repair, and as the body can't produce vitamin C, you do have to get it from your diet. If that means eating butternut squash occasionally I'm okay with that. I'd start with this recipe right here.

Preheat the oven to 200°C fan/220°C conventional/gas mark 7.

Drizzle the squash halves with olive oil and roast in the oven for around 30 minutes, until cooked through. Meanwhile, cook the quinoa in a pan of salted water as per the packet instructions, putting half a lemon into the pan, too.

Roughly chop the feta, sundried tomatoes and spinach leaves into chickpea-sized pieces. Drain and rinse the chickpeas. Add all of these to the cooked quinoa and stir well. Remove the lemon half from the cooked quinoa.

Season with salt and pepper and juice from the remaining half a lemon. Once the squash is ready, spoon the filling on top and serve.

TIP Scoop out some extra squash from each half to make room for more filling and save it for another salad or use it in place of sweet potato in another recipe.

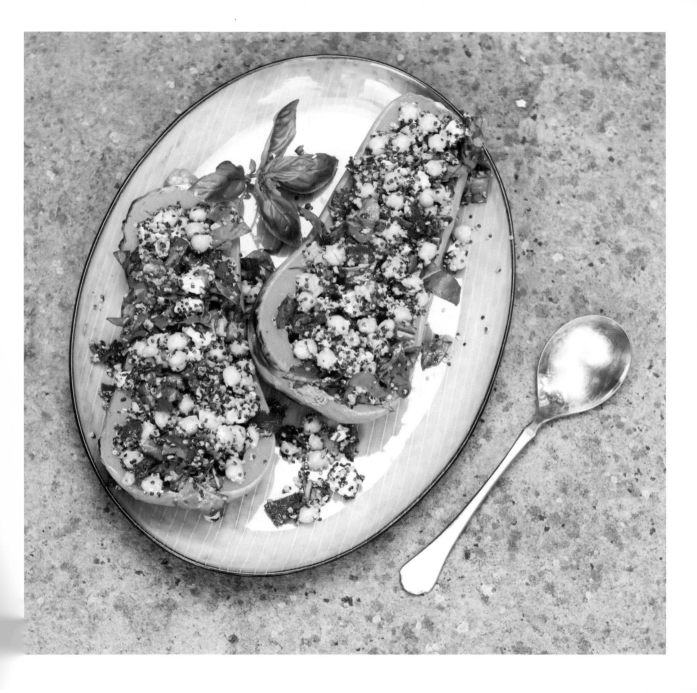

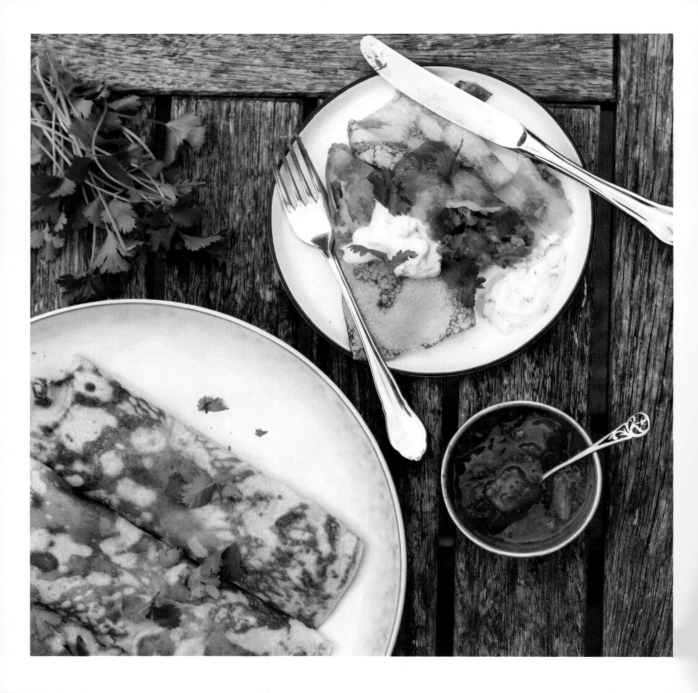

SWEET POTATO MASALA DOSA

MAKES 6

- 100g gram flour
- 100g plain flour
- 200ml milk (any kind)
- Salt
- 750g sweet potatoes
- Vegetable oil
- 1 onion (around 100g), peeled and finely diced
- 4 garlic cloves
- 1 tbsp ground ginger or 4cm piece of fresh ginger, grated
- Small bunch of fresh coriander, leaves picked and stalks finely chopped
- 2 tsp ground turmeric
- 1 tsp ground coriander
- 1 tsp garam masala

Good old onions and garlic again. Have you noticed they've become a bit of a theme in this chapter? They are pretty damn amazing though, and the vitamin A-loaded sweet potatoes (an antioxidant) certainly won't do your liver any harm either. If you've never had a dosa before, you're in for a treat!

Preheat the oven to 200°C fan/220°C conventional/gas mark 7.

Mix together the flours, milk, a pinch of salt and 300ml of water and set aside. This will be your dosa batter.

Peel the sweet potato and chop into cubes, then drizzle with oil and salt and roast in the oven for 20–30 minutes, until nicely cooked through.

Heat a glug of vegetable oil in a large frying pan. Add the onion and peel and crush the garlic cloves into the pan. Fry for 5 minutes.

Add the ginger, chopped coriander stalks, turmeric and ground coriander and stir for another minute. Add 100ml of water and stir.

Once cooked, add the sweet potato to the pan and mash roughly, though not completely.

Add the garam masala and coriander leaves and season to taste. Transfer this filling to a bowl.>

SWEET POTATO MASALA DOSA cont.

Clean the pan and heat a small amount of oil, using a piece of kitchen towel to spread it around the pan.

Add a ladleful of the dosa batter so it just reaches the edges of the pan. Once it has almost cooked on top, place a large spoonful of the sweet potato filling in a line in the centre.

When the dosa is nice and brown and crisp underneath, use a spatula to gently fold one side of the dosa over the mixture and roll it in the pan (like wrapping a very hot fajita), so that the join is facing down into the pan. Cook for another minute before transferring to a plate.

Repeat this for each dosa, keeping them warm by placing the plate in a low oven between batches.

 TIP Serve with Indian chutneys and raita for those who like it less spicy.

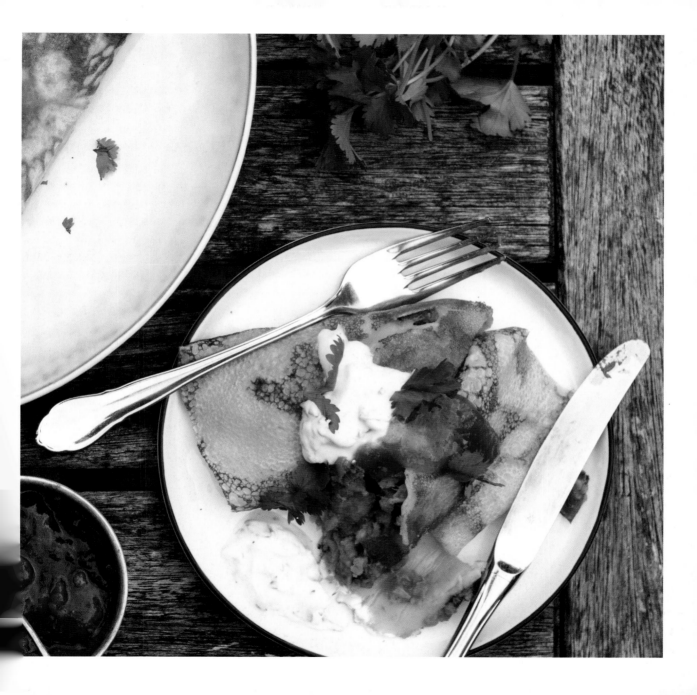

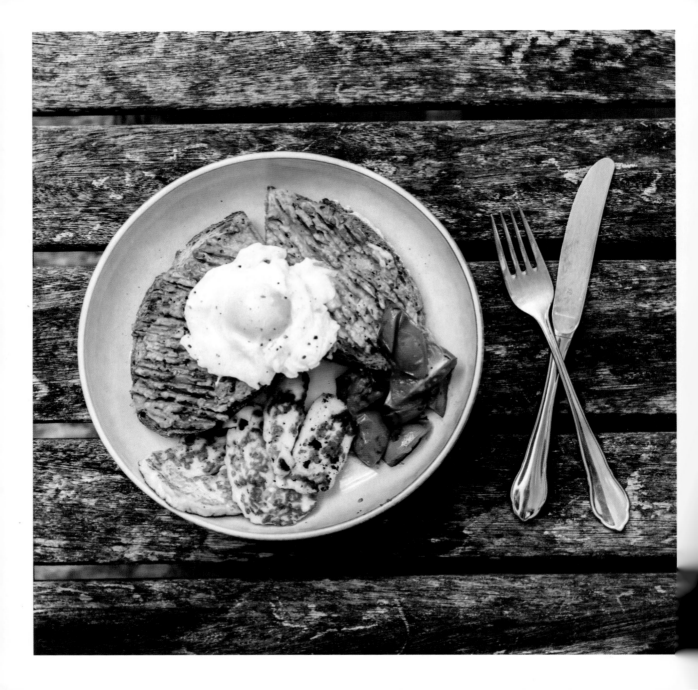

ULTIMATE VEGGIE BRUNCH

SERVES 1

- 1 slice of sourdough bread
- Olive oil
- 80g tomatoes
- ½ large avocado
- Salt and pepper
- 3 slices of halloumi
- 1–2 medium eggs
- Coffee!

If you have a hangover and need to 'detox' your body of alcohol, this brunch should be top of your list of foods to eat. While there's nothing that can really speed up the process of metabolising alcohol except time, giving your body all the building blocks it needs to do that certainly helps. Here we have carbohydrates from the bread, fats from the avocado and halloumi, protein from the eggs and lycopene from the tomatoes. Lycopene is the phytochemical and antioxidant that makes tomatoes red and keeps your liver happy.

Get ready to multitask: place a large frying pan over a medium heat, bring a small saucepan of water to the boil and prepare your coffee.

Toast the bread.

Drizzle a little olive oil on one side of the frying pan.

Roughly chop the tomatoes and add them to that side.

Mash the avocado on the toast and season with salt and pepper.

Turn down the heat under the frying pan and add the halloumi to the other side of the pan. Cook for a few minutes on each side.

Crack the egg(s) into the boiling water and poach for 3 minutes, until the white is opaque.

Assemble everything on a plate and tuck in immediately.

Fats

THE 'FATS ARE BAD' MYTH

We like a simple solution when it comes to nutrition: a single food to eat for good health or a single way of eating to cure or prevent everything. It's a narrative that we heavily lean towards. After a while, you tend to see a pattern with weight-loss diets: high carb low fat, then low carb high fat, repeat until the end of time. The same concept comes around time and time again, just repackaged under a different name. In the 80s, we were convinced that fat was the cause of all problems, and this narrative has shaped our food choices since.

So, let's talk fats.

Fat plays a huge variety of roles in the body. Every cell in the body is encased by a lipid cell membrane, which contains fats and cholesterol, and helps control what goes in and out of each cell. Your nerve cells have an additional coating called myelin, which improves electrical signalling. On a larger scale, fats are important for insulation, protecting vital organs, providing a protective barrier on your skin and starting chemical reactions to control growth and immune functions. Fat-soluble vitamins are stored in the liver, and your sex hormones are made from cholesterol. Basically, you need fat to live.

FATS AND HEART HEALTH

Many people will have had blood tests to check their cholesterol levels. I myself have had many of them. If you haven't yet, prepare yourself for what's to come later in life. Cholesterol is made by the body and regulated by the liver, but it can also be obtained from the diet. When you have your cholesterol levels checked, your results show the levels of low-density lipoprotein (LDL), high-density lipoprotein (HDL) and triglycerides (dietary fat) in your blood. I'm going to use the terms triglycerides and fats interchangeably for the sake of simplicity.

Lipoproteins are complex particles with a protein coat on the outside and lipids (fats) in the centre (hence lipo-protein). We need them to carry fats around the body as blood is a water-based fluid, and water and fat don't mix. There are five groups of lipoproteins: chylomicrons, VLDL, LDL, HDL and IDL. They all transport fats in the bloodstream.

• Chylomicrons and VLDLs deliver fats to various cells in the body.

• LDLs deliver cholesterol to cells in the body.

• HDLs take excess cholesterol from the body and transport it back to the liver to either be recycled or eliminated from the body.

One of the reasons LDLs have been linked to heart disease is because of a genetic condition called familial hypercholesterolaemia (FH). People with FH have very high blood LDL levels and have a greater risk of heart disease at a younger age. The high level of LDLs in the blood occur due to a genetic fault, rather than lifestyle.

High LDL levels are linked to atherosclerosis and heart disease, but the exact cause of atherosclerosis is not known. It is suspected that it begins with damage to the artery wall lining, which means that LDLs can then enter the wall and become trapped, forming a plaque. We know that plaques are made of fat, cholesterol, calcium and other substances, and that they harden over time and cause arteries to narrow. If an artery blocks completely, it can lead to a heart attack or stroke.

This is why LDL is seen as 'bad' cholesterol and HDL, which removes excess cholesterol from the body, is seen as 'good'. In reality we need a little of both, with more HDL than LDL. Overall, having high LDL, low HDL and high triglyceride levels produces the highest risk for heart disease [1]. So how does this relate to our diet?

Dietary fats have an effect on blood LDL levels, and therefore on the risk of heart disease. Trans fats have a negative effect and increase risk, whereas unsaturated fats have a beneficial effect and decrease risk [2]. (Tip: if any of these terms seem unfamiliar, check back to Chapter 2 and the section on fats!)

Trans fats are formed when oil is hydrogenated, which hardens it. Trans fats are consistently associated with increased risk of heart disease [3], as they increase LDL, decrease HDL and increase triglyceride levels. They also promote inflammation. Luckily, trans fats have been massively reduced in the UK, with supermarkets removing them from all products in 2007, and many businesses also removing or drastically reducing them in their products.

Notice I didn't mention saturated fat earlier; that's because I think placing it in the same category as trans fats too easily feeds into the simple narrative of 'unsaturated = good' and 'saturated = bad', when it's a little more nuanced than that. Saturated fat in itself isn't inherently bad for us, it depends on context. Before you misunderstand me: a diet that contains high amounts of saturated fat as a percentage of overall energy intake is linked to increased risk of heart disease. Evidence shows that reducing intake of saturated fat as a proportion of overall fat intake (but not reducing total fat) has beneficial effects [4], but what we replace it with matters: replacing with unsaturated fats had a much more positive effect than replacing with simple carbohydrates (i.e. sugars).

Notice that none of the research involves cutting out saturated fat entirely,

PIXIE TIP
If any of the terms in this chapter seem unfamiliar, check back to Chapter 2 and the section on fats.

because it's pretty impossible to do. We like to group foods by fat type: avocado – unsaturated, cheese – saturated, when in fact even foods like avocados and olive oil contain some saturated fat. You can't avoid it, it's in pretty much every food that has fat! This is why we have recommendations that state saturated fat intake should ideally be less than 10% of our daily energy intake. In the context of an overall diet, where saturated fat is a smaller component of total fat intake than unsaturated fat, it's completely fine.

Pretty much all foods with fat contain a mixture of saturated and unsaturated – even avocados.

It's also important to note that we don't eat these nutrients in isolation, and so the source of these fats does make a difference. For example, if you eat a piece of cheese then yes, you're eating some saturated fat, but you're also getting protein and calcium. In fact, some evidence shows that dairy doesn't increase your risk of heart disease, but also doesn't decrease it either, so it's pretty neutral [5]. Eating a piece of cheese is very different to eating a large meat feast pizza, which contains several sources of saturated fat and probably more than you should ideally be consuming in a single day. Having one of those once in a blue moon won't hurt you, but having one every day would probably increase your risk of heart disease.

By replacing some of the saturated fats in our diet with unsaturated fats, we can decrease our risk of developing heart disease [4, 5], particularly if our diet happens to contain a larger proportion of saturated fats. This can be as simple as substituting olive oil for butter in a recipe.

There is a plausible mechanism by which a diet high in saturated fat raises blood LDL levels and increases risk of heart disease. Seems like a straightforward scientific consensus, and it is, but those in the low carb, anti-sugar camp are not happy. They have rallied against the American Heart Association lately, blaming their conclusions that we should aim for a lower saturated fat intake on them having a bias against fat since the 1980s. But I don't think that's justified, as the AHA are not alone in their reasoning; many independent experts and boards have come to the same conclusion based on the evidence available. Call me cynical, but if you're promoting a low carb high fat diet, then of course you don't want the evidence to show that any fat leads to heart disease.

We used to think that cholesterol intake increased the risk of heart disease, but that isn't so clear-cut. For example, although egg yolks contain cholesterol, egg consumption is not associated with heart disease risk [6]. The low carb brigade likes to take this uncertainty and 'change of heart' (which, by the way, has only occurred due to new evidence) and use it as proof that we're also completely wrong about saturated fat, which is missing the point. New studies on saturated fat are being conducted every year, and yet the consensus still holds, because the majority of evidence still supports the consensus. That's how science works.

There is research showing that a low carbohydrate diet neither increases nor decreases LDL cholesterol [7], but this fails to acknowledge that it's not ALL fat that increases risk, just high amounts of saturated fat, and although you may assume that a low carb diet is high in saturated fats, it isn't necessarily. There was also significant weight loss in participants, which is known to reduce both LDL cholesterol and the risk of heart disease.

I'm by no means saying that we have to reduce our overall fat intake and go for a low fat diet, not at all. In fact, the Mediterranean diet, which is widely agreed upon to be an incredibly healthy dietary pattern, is neither a low fat nor a high fat diet; it's simply a moderate fat diet and includes some saturated fat such as cheese. This just goes to show that a whole-diet approach is more important than saying 'unsaturated fats are good, saturated fats are bad'.

A whole-diet approach is more important than simply saying 'unsaturated fats = good, saturated = bad'.

THE COCONUT OIL MYTH

Seeing as we're on the subject of saturated fat, it would be a shame not to go off on a quick tangent about coconut oil. Especially as the many health claims surrounding it are almost too numerous and stupid to mention.

Coconut oil is around 85% saturated fat, most of which is lauric acid. Despite this, it has somehow reached 'superfood' status, thanks to some clever marketing tactics. Coconut oil has celebrity (and wellness blogger) endorsement, exaggerated scientific claims that give it the illusion of credibility, appeal to nature (it's just so unprocessed), and a feel of the exotic about it that reminds you of happier times lying on a beach somewhere.

Coconut oil isn't 'special' in terms of the effects its saturated fat content has on heart disease risk. The evidence 'does not support popular claims purporting that coconut oil is a healthy oil in terms of reducing the risk of CVD' (heart disease)[8].

A lot of the claims around coconut oil are extrapolated from research into medium chain triglycerides (MCTs). These are saturated fatty acids with 6–10 carbons. Lauric acid, the main component of coconut oil, has 12 carbons, and so isn't considered a 'true' MCT [9] as it behaves differently in the body, which is also why MCT oil doesn't contain lauric acid. With that in mind, coconut oil therefore actually only contains around 5–10% MCTs, so it's a bit of a stretch to apply the benefits of MCTs to coconut oil. And there are some benefits. MCTs are described as 'fat-burning fat' as they are quickly metabolised for energy rather than stored. They also raise HDL levels. All good stuff but coconut oil contains so few MCTs, it can hardly lay claim to these benefits.

Coconut oil is neither 'good' nor 'bad', but shouldn't be consumed in excess. It is a saturated fat, and as such I can't, in good faith, recommend putting it in your coffee every morning as many wellness bloggers do. Same goes for butter for that matter; I mean not only does it sound absolutely vile, it's not going to offer you amazing health benefits either. Coconut oil is a great make-up remover though, I'll give it that much.

UNSATURATED FATS – THE 'HEALTHY' FATS?

So enough about saturated fats, what about the unsaturated ones?

Unsaturated fats are seen as the good guys. They're the 'healthy fats' you've probably seen people mention in passing on Instagram, when they probably don't themselves know what they mean by 'healthy fats'. Unsaturated fats can be mono- or polyunsaturated, and are found in foods like vegetable oils, nuts, avocado and oily fish.

First, let's quickly talk about inflammation. Inflammation occurs in response to injury, bacterial infection, or other trauma, such as an allergy. You experience heat, redness, swelling, pain and loss of function. Your arteries dilate to increase blood flow, and white blood cells move to the area to ingest any foreign material, bringing fluid with them, which is what causes the swelling. Think of the last time you had a burn or cut. You'll likely have experienced some if not all of these symptoms. Your body's normal inflammatory response is vital. The aim of inflammation is to kill, dilute, wall-off, and prepare the tissue for wound healing. This is then followed by an anti-inflammatory response. Problems arise when there is too much inflammation or too little inflammation.

Broadly speaking, omega-3 fatty acids are seen as anti-inflammatory whereas omega-6 fatty acids are seen as inflammatory. This concept is not particularly helpful though, as again, it's not that simple. Both omega-3 and omega-6 intakes are associated with lower inflammatory markers, and both have

PIXIE TIP
Both omega-3 and omega-6 have anti-inflammatory effects.

119

The more
refined an oil is,
the higher the
smoke point, as
there are fewer
impurities.

anti-inflammatory effects, although omega-3 more so than omega-6. Both higher omega-3 and higher omega-6 intakes are also associated with reduced heart disease risk [10].

As a population, we get decent amounts of omega-6 in our diet already from vegetable oils and olive oil, but we could probably do with a bit more omega-3. Good ways to get this are flaxseed, walnuts and oily fish. This does not mean that omega-6 is 'bad' or that vegetable oils are 'bad' for you and you need to avoid them. The idea of an 'anti-inflammatory diet' is a bit redundant as this is easily achieved by simply eating a balanced diet, which can easily include vegetable oils.

Funnily enough, in the wellness blogosphere, extra virgin olive oil is seen as a 'healthy' oil to use, whereas vegetable oils are not. But most vegetable oils found in supermarkets consist entirely (or at least mostly) of rapeseed oil (also known as canola oil), which has higher levels of omega-3 than olive oil. Rapeseed and vegetable oils in general are demonised for being 'processed', but all oils are processed in one way or another. Contrary to what scaremongers will tell you, rapeseed oil is associated with a whole host of health benefits [11], including lowering cholesterol and improving insulin sensitivity.

SMOKING HOT OILS

The smoke point is the temperature at which an oil starts to burn and smoke. Going past the smoke point gives food a burnt flavour, destroys beneficial phytochemicals and makes it prone to oxidation, which is a process that changes the chemical structure of the oil, thereby potentially producing harmful compounds.

When you pan-fry something, the temperature doesn't tend to go above around 120°C, whereas in an oven it obviously depends on the oven temperature. The more refined an oil is, the higher the smoke point, as there are less impurities. But smoke points also depend on other factors such as the volume of oil and the size of the pan used.

I commonly see people say not to cook with extra virgin olive oil and to only use it in dressings due to its low smoke point, but that's unnecessary. Extra virgin olive oil has a smoke point of between 160–200°C, so it's perfectly fine to cook with. In fact, depending on the type, olive oil can actually have a higher smoke point than coconut oil. So please don't stress about which oil to cook with – go with what will taste best and what you have on hand. The only one I wouldn't recommend cooking with is flaxseed oil, as that has a very low smoke point. Save that one for the dressings.

THE GREAT SUGAR VS FAT DEBATE

Many fad diets have been born out of the notion that there is a perfect macro-nutrient ratio, and the low carb vs low fat argument has been raging on for what seems like forever. Here's where it comes back to weight again, because we generally measure the success of a diet based on weight loss rather than health gain.

It's convenient and simple to believe that a single nutrient is the cause of all chronic health problems. As you can hopefully appreciate by now, it's never that simple, and even within macronutrients not all fats and not all carbs will behave the same way in the body. Reducing all fats doesn't make sense as mono- and polyunsaturated fats have such beneficial effects, and reducing all carbs doesn't make sense either as whole grains have amazingly beneficial fibre.

Decades ago, public health guidelines told us to reduce our saturated fat intake, yet rates of obesity and metabolic syndrome continued to rise. Metabolic syndrome is a collection of conditions that occur together – including increased blood pressure, high blood sugar, and abnormal blood cholesterol or triglyceride levels – which increase the risk of developing heart disease and type 2 diabetes. Next, it was decided sugar was to blame, and it was assumed that telling people to reduce their saturated fat intake meant we were eating more simple carbohydrates (sometimes true but not always). Yet even though sugar consumption has been dropping in the UK since 1992, obesity rates are still on the rise [12]. If sugar really is to blame, how can this be the case? Well obviously, it's not to blame. Sugar has been shown to NOT be uniquely related to weight gain or metabolic syndrome [13]. Replacing sugar with other macronutrients, but keeping total calorie intake the same, has no effect on body weight. Sugar may be a contributor, but it's not the sole cause.

The same people who said we were stupid for believing a single nutrient (saturated fat) could cause all our problems are often now the same people blaming a single nutrient (sugar) for all our problems. Great! Makes total sense. Glad we all learnt our lesson there.

Low fat, low carb or somewhere in between, do whatever works for you. Just don't act like because it suits you, it'll suit everyone. I'm all for a middle ground. I like the message of moderation, like in the Mediterranean diet, and the following recipes will definitely reflect that. I've used sources of saturated fat, especially cheese, as a bit of cheese is nothing to be afraid of. I also really love cheese, and couldn't resist including all my favourites. Of course, there are plenty of sources of unsaturated fats there too!

The same people who said we were stupid for believing a single nutrient (saturated fat) could cause all our problems are often now the same people blaming a single nutrient (sugar) for all our problems. Glad we all learnt our lesson there

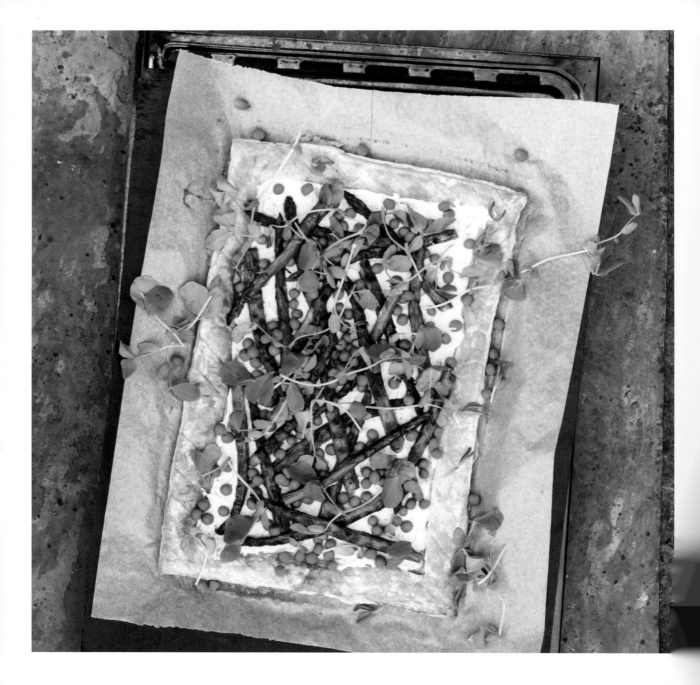

ASPARAGUS & PEA TART

SERVES 4

- 1 ready rolled puff pastry sheet (320g)
- 1 medium egg, beaten
- 250g ricotta
- ½ lemon, zested and juiced
- 1 tbsp olive oil, plus extra for drizzling
- 1 small garlic clove
- Sprig of fresh mint
- Sprig of fresh basil
- Salt and pepper
- 500g asparagus, woody ends removed
- 100g frozen peas
- 50g pea shoots

Ricotta isn't the most interesting of cheeses, but it tastes brilliant when paired with lemon, garlic and herbs. It contains saturated fats, yes, but that's not a reason you can't enjoy it in moderation, especially with such delicious vegetables!

Preheat the oven to 180°C fan/200°C conventional/gas mark 6. Line a flat surface with baking paper and unroll the pastry. Score a 2cm border around the edge and brush the surface with the beaten egg. Transfer the pastry on the baking paper to a baking tray and bake for around 15 minutes, until puffed up and golden.

Blend the ricotta, lemon juice and zest, oil, garlic, mint and basil in a blender or food processor until smooth. Season and adjust to taste.

Bring a medium saucepan of salted water to the boil. Add the asparagus and cook for 3 minutes (skip this stage if you have very fine asparagus or if you like very crunchy asparagus).

Place the cooked asparagus on a hot griddle pan. Drizzle with olive oil and cook on all sides. Add the peas to the asparagus water and cook for 3 minutes, or until they bob to the surface.

Remove the pastry from the oven and gently press down the middle rectangle, leaving the border puffed up. Spread the ricotta mixture evenly over the centre, then place the asparagus on top followed by the peas. Sprinkle with pea shoots before serving.

AUBERGINE HALLOUMI ROLLS

SERVES 2

- 1 aubergine (around 300g)
- Olive oil
- Salt and pepper
- 200g halloumi
- Small handful of fresh basil leaves, one per roll
- 50g salad leaves
- 100g tomatoes
- 1 tbsp rapeseed oil
- 1 tbsp balsamic vinegar

Halloumi is one of my favourite cheeses (doesn't everyone have a favourite cheese?), but it does go rubbery if you let it cool after cooking, so eat it quickly! As mentioned before, the saturated fat in cheese may be pretty neutral when it comes to heart disease, and context matters. By pairing it with ingredients such as aubergine, basil, oil and tomatoes, it's a great Mediterranean-style meal!

Preheat the oven to 200°C fan/220°C conventional/gas mark 7.

Slice the aubergine lengthways around 5mm thick. Heat a griddle pan and brush with olive oil. Grill the aubergine slices on both sides, seasoning with a little salt and pepper on each side. Set to one side to cool.

Slice the halloumi and cook on the griddle pan for a few minutes each side, then set aside.

Place a piece of halloumi on each aubergine slice with a basil leaf, then roll up roughly and place on a lined baking tray. Repeat this for each slice. Bake in the oven for 10 minutes.

In the meantime, make a salad with the leaves and tomatoes and any other items you desire, and divide it between two plates. Place a few of the aubergine halloumi rolls on each plate when ready to serve. Drizzle with rapeseed oil and balsamic vinegar.

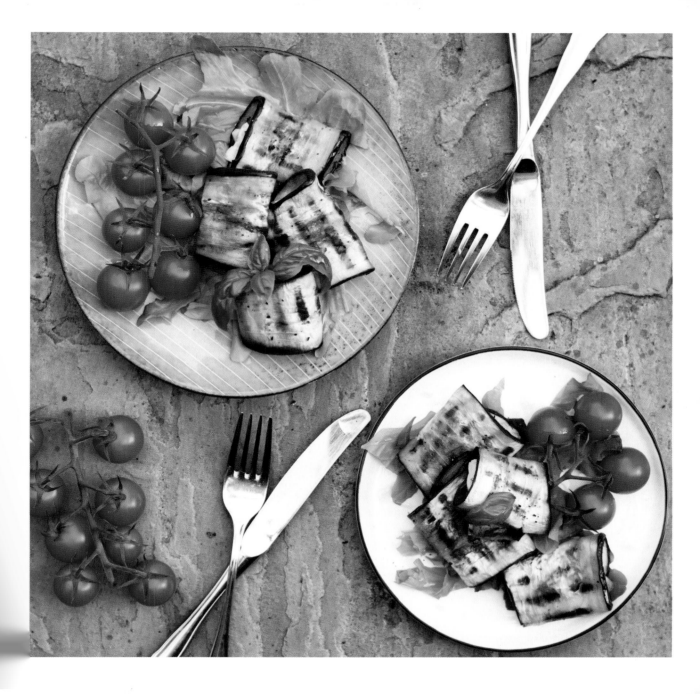

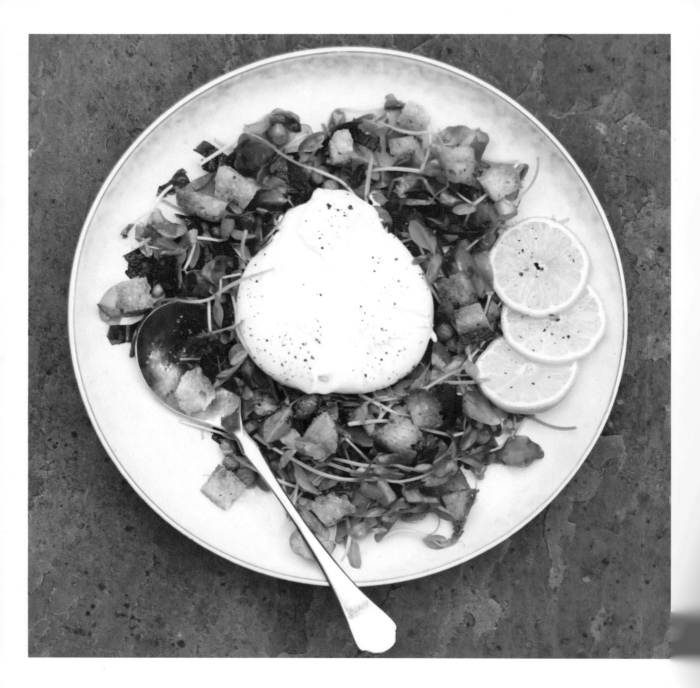

BURRATA, PEA & MINT SALAD

SERVES 3-4

- 1 slice of sourdough bread
- Olive oil
- Salt and pepper
- 100g frozen peas
- 50g pea shoots
- 1 tbsp fresh mint leaves, finely chopped
- Lemon juice
- 200g burrata (undrained weight)

Burrata is the king of cheeses. It's pure perfection and deserves to be the centrepiece of a dish. Combining it with greens gives this meal a perfect balance, and yes, that includes the saturated fat in the cheese.

Set the oven to grill or preheat to 200°C fan/220°C conventional/ gas mark 6.

Cut the sourdough into cubes, place on a lined baking tray and drizzle with olive oil, salt and pepper.

Grill for around 5-10 minutes or bake until the cubes are nicely crisped up like croutons.

In the meantime, bring a saucepan of water to the boil and cook the peas for 5 minutes.

Toss the pea shoots and mint together and drizzle with a little olive oil and lemon juice. Place the leaves on a large serving plate.

Once cooked, add the peas and croutons. Or leave them to cool first if you prefer.

Finally, carefully place the burrata on top, drizzle with olive oil and more lemon juice and season with salt and pepper.

FETA PARCELS WITH TZATZIKI

MAKES 12 PARCELS

- 200g spinach leaves
- 100g feta
- 2 spring onions, finely sliced
- 1 tsp dried or fresh oregano
- 1 tsp dried or fresh basil
- Salt and pepper
- 3 sheets of filo pastry
- Olive oil

For the tzatziki
- 80g cucumber
- 1 garlic clove
- 1 tbsp fresh or 1 tsp dried mint leaves
- 200g plain yoghurt
- 1 tbsp lemon juice

This chapter has essentially turned into an ode to cheese, which is perfectly fine by me. After all, pretty much all Mediterranean cultures eat cheese. These bite-sized parcels are quick, simple and delicious!

Preheat the oven to 200 fan/220°C conventional/gas mark 6.

Chop the spinach and wilt it slightly in a large saucepan with a little bit of water. Remove any excess water.

Crumble the feta into a bowl. Add the spring onions, wilted spinach, oregano and basil. Season with salt and pepper.

Cut a sheet of filo pastry in half, then in half again. You should have four strips, each of which needs to be folded in half to make four squares. Brush each pastry square with olive oil on both sides.

Place a heaped tablespoon of the feta mixture on the centre of each pastry square. Take the corners and scrunch up in the middle, then place on a lined baking tray. Repeat this for each of the four squares. Repeat steps 3–4 for the other two sheets.

Bake the parcels in the oven for 12 minutes. In the meantime, make the tzatziki: grate the cucumber, peel and crush the garlic and finely chop the mint. Mix together the yoghurt, cucumber, lemon juice, garlic and chopped mint. Season with salt and pepper.

When the filo parcels are ready, serve with the tzatziki.

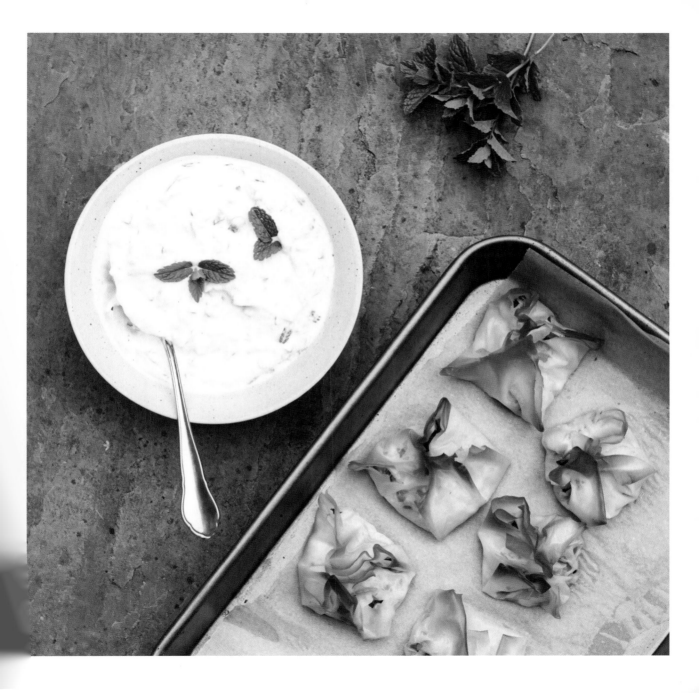

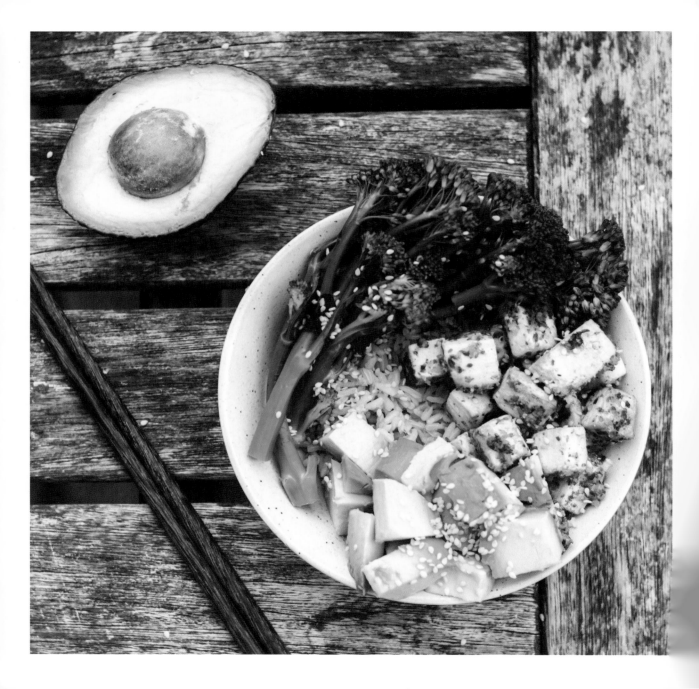

FLAXSEED-CRUSTED TOFU BOWL

SERVES 1

- 100g firm tofu
- 2 tbsp lemon juice
- 2 tbsp light soy sauce
- 60g brown rice
- 10g fresh or dried breadcrumbs
- 10g ground flaxseed
- Sesame or olive oil
- 80g tenderstem broccoli
- ½ avocado, cubed
- Sesame seeds, toasted

Don't eat fish but want omega-3? Have some flaxseed. Add it to your smoothies, sprinkle it on your cereal or use it to elevate your tofu to the next level. No bland tofu here!

If the tofu isn't firm, press it by wrapping it up and placing something heavy on top for 10 minutes.

Cut the tofu into cubes, then place into a shallow bowl with 1 tablespoon of the lemon juice and 1 tablespoon of the soy sauce mixed together. Leave to marinate for 10 minutes.

Cook the brown rice in boiling water mixed with the remaining lemon juice and soy sauce according to the packet instructions.

Mix together the breadcrumbs and ground flaxseed in a bowl. Toss the tofu in the mixture until well coated.

Heat a glug of oil in a large frying pan and fry the tofu gently, turning occasionally to cook on all sides.

Steam the broccoli for 5 minutes or boil for 3 minutes.

To assemble the bowl, fill the bottom with warm brown rice, then place the broccoli, tofu and avocado on top. Drizzle over any remaining marinade and sprinkle with toasted sesame seeds.

LENTIL, FIG & AVOCADO SALAD WITH TAHINI DRESSING

SERVES 2

- 4 fresh figs
- 1 avocado
- 200g cooked puy lentils (100g raw)
- 50g rocket

For the dressing
- 2 tbsp tahini
- ¼ tsp salt
- ¼ tsp garlic granules or powder

Avocado is the ultimate 'healthy fats' champion. I don't think I've ever heard someone claim that avocados are bad for you, and that's saying something! Avocados are rich in unsaturated fats as well as containing vitamin E.

Cut the figs into quarters and the avocado into cubes.

Mix together the cooked lentils, figs, avocado and rocket in a serving bowl.

Mix together the tahini, salt and garlic granules or powder with 3 tablespoons of water.

Drizzle the dressing over the salad and serve.

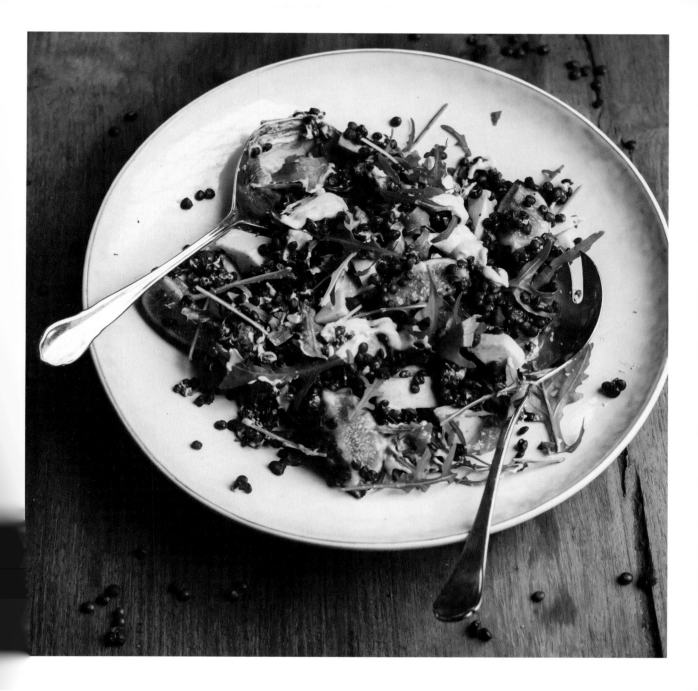

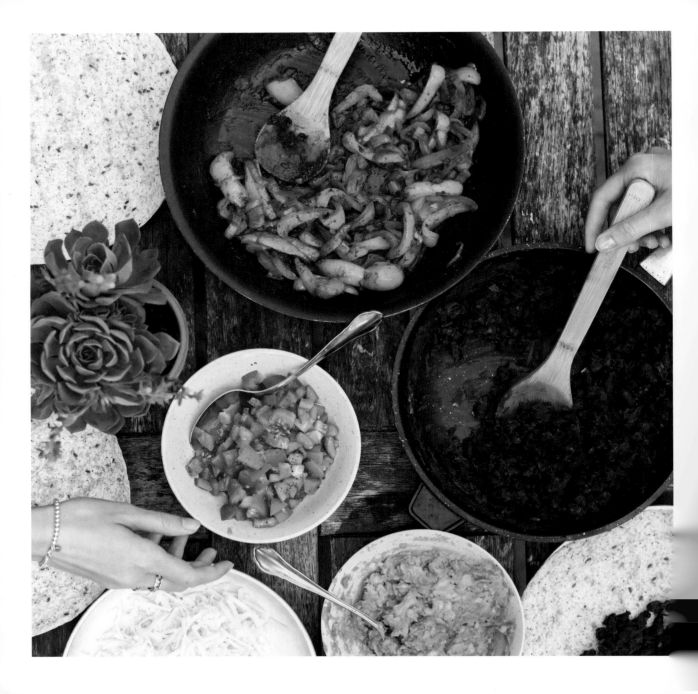

MEXICAN FEAST

SERVES 4

- Olive oil
- 1 large onion (around 150g), peeled and sliced
- 1 orange pepper, sliced
- 1 yellow pepper, sliced
- 1 x 400g tin of black beans, drained and rinsed
- 1 x 400g tin of kidney beans, drained and rinsed
- 2 tbsp fajita spice mix (or make your own, see below)
- 250g cheddar cheese, grated
- 200g tomatoes
- 2 large avocados
- 50g salad leaves of choice, chopped
- Salt and pepper
- ½ lemon, juiced
- 8 tortillas

Whether you're into cheese or not, by cooking the beans and vegetables in this dish with olive oil, you're getting some heart-healthy monounsaturated fats with every mouthful!

Heat a glug of olive oil in a large frying pan over a medium heat. Add the onion and cook for 5 minutes before adding the peppers. Add about 50ml of water and let it simmer until the water has all gone.

Heat another glug of oil in a saucepan over a medium-low heat and add the beans. Stir for a minute, then add about 50ml of water and let it simmer until the water has all gone. Season the beans and the peppers with 1 tablespoon of fajita seasoning each. Add a little more water if needed to avoid things sticking to the bottom of the pan.

To make the salsa, season the tomato with salt, pepper and a little lemon juice. Set aside. To make the guacamole: mash the avocados in a bowl and season with salt, pepper and a little lemon juice. Set aside.

Put the salad leaves in a bowl. When the beans and peppers are ready, remove from the heat and pour into two serving dishes. Put the beans, peppers, tomato salsa, guacamole, cheese and salad on the table. Warm the tortillas in the microwave for 30 seconds and let everyone assemble their own perfect fajita.

TIP To make your own fajita seasoning, mix together 1 tsp onion powder, 1 tsp garlic granules or powder, 1 tsp paprika, 1 tsp cumin, 1 tsp salt and 1 tsp mild chilli powder.

MUSHROOMY MACARONI CHEESE

SERVES 2-3

- 150g dried pasta (macaroni or penne are best)
- 1 tbsp olive oil
- 2 heaped tbsp plain flour
- 350ml milk (any kind)
- 2 garlic cloves
- 200g white or brown mushrooms, sliced
- Salt and pepper
- 150g cheddar cheese, grated
- 20g Parmesan, grated

This recipe is dedicated to my sister Emily, whose love for macaroni cheese is slightly ironic considering too much dairy gives her digestive problems. Here we have cheddar and Parmesan cheese - a double whammy of deliciousness!

Cook the pasta in a large saucepan of salted water for 2 minutes less than packet instructions.

In a separate saucepan, heat the olive oil, then stir in the flour. Slowly whisk in the milk a little at a time, making sure any lumps are quickly removed.

Peel and crush the garlic and add to the sauce with the sliced mushrooms. Simmer gently over a low heat for 15 minutes.

Remove the pan from the heat and season the sauce with salt and pepper, then add most (but not all) of the cheddar. Stir until smooth.

Add the pasta to the sauce, mix together and pour into an ovenproof dish. Sprinkle the rest of the cheddar and all of the Parmesan on top.

Set the oven to grill and, when hot, grill the dish for about 5-10 minutes, until brown and crispy on top. Serve hot!

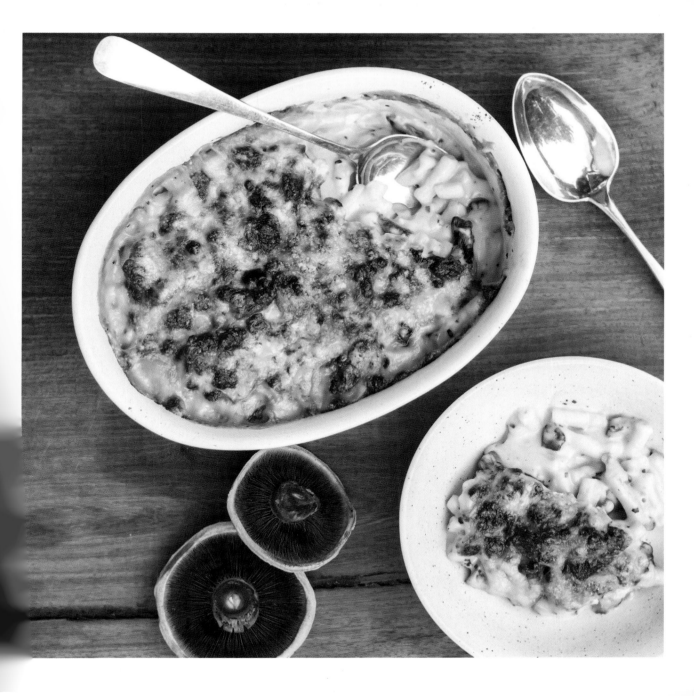

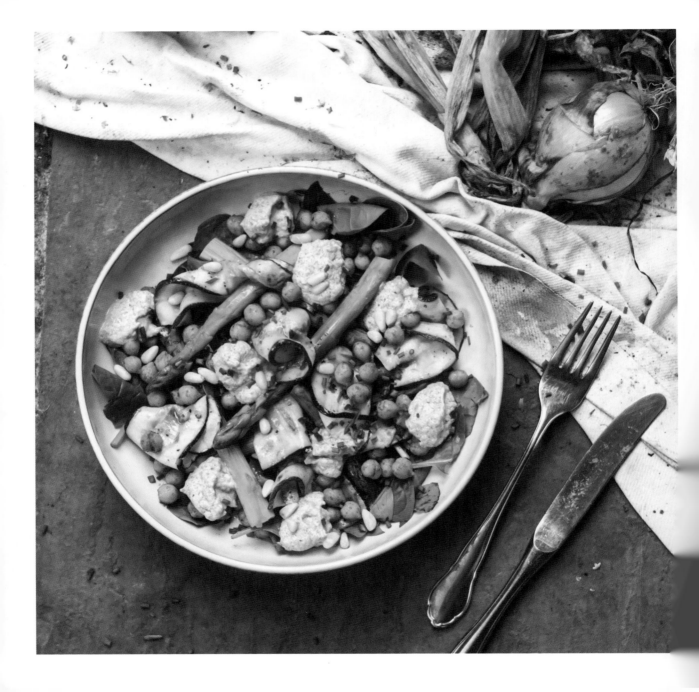

ASPARAGUS SALAD WITH CHICKPEAS & YOGHURT DRESSING

SERVES 2-3

- 1 courgette (around 200g)
- Olive oil
- Salt and pepper
- 250g asparagus
- 1 x 400g tin of chickpeas, drained and rinsed
- Paprika
- 50g salad leaves
- 10g pine nuts
- 150g Greek yoghurt
- 150g aubergine pesto (if you can't get hold of this, then follow the yoghurt dip from the roasted aubergine recipe on page 235)

Nuts are a great source of unsaturated fats, as well as fat-soluble vitamins like vitamin E. They make a great snack, but also taste great when sprinkled on salads like this one!

Cut the courgette lengthways into long, thin slices. Place in a microwaveable bowl, cover, and cook for 3 minutes on high.

Heat a little olive oil in a griddle pan on high heat, grill the courgette ribbons, sprinkling a little salt and pepper on both sides, and set aside.

Cook the asparagus by boiling or steaming for 5 minutes and set aside.

Put the chickpeas into a saucepan on medium heat with a little olive oil, salt and a pinch of paprika. Cook for around 5 minutes.

If you prefer, let the vegetables and chickpeas cool.

Assemble the salad: create a bed of salad leaves, add the asparagus and chickpeas, artfully (or not) place the courgette slices on top and sprinkle with pine nuts.

Mix the yoghurt and aubergine pesto together and dollop on top to serve.

TEX-MEX EGGS

SERVES 2

- 250g sweet potato, peeled and cubed
- Olive oil
- 1 onion (around 80-100g), peeled and finely diced
- 1 tsp paprika
- 1 tsp ground cumin
- 1 x 400g tin of black beans, drained and rinsed
- 2 tbsp tomato purée
- Salt and pepper
- 1 lime
- 4 medium eggs
- 1 avocado, sliced

Eggs once had a bad rep, but now that we know the cholesterol in egg yolks isn't linked to increased risk of heart disease, you can enjoy this delicious meal without worrying about it!

Put the sweet potato cubes into a microwaveable bowl, cover, and microwave for 6-8 minutes on high, until soft.

Heat a glug of olive oil in a large frying pan over a medium heat and fry the diced onion for 5 minutes. Add the spices and beans to the pan along with a splash of water. Cook for 2 minutes.

Add the sweet potato and tomato purée and cook for another 2 minutes. Season with salt, pepper and lime juice.

Make four wells in the saucepan and crack in the eggs.

Add a lid if possible and cook over a low heat for around 8 minutes, until the egg whites are just cooked and the yolks are runny. If you're not a fan of runny eggs, then cook for around 12 minutes.

Place the avocado slices on top to serve.

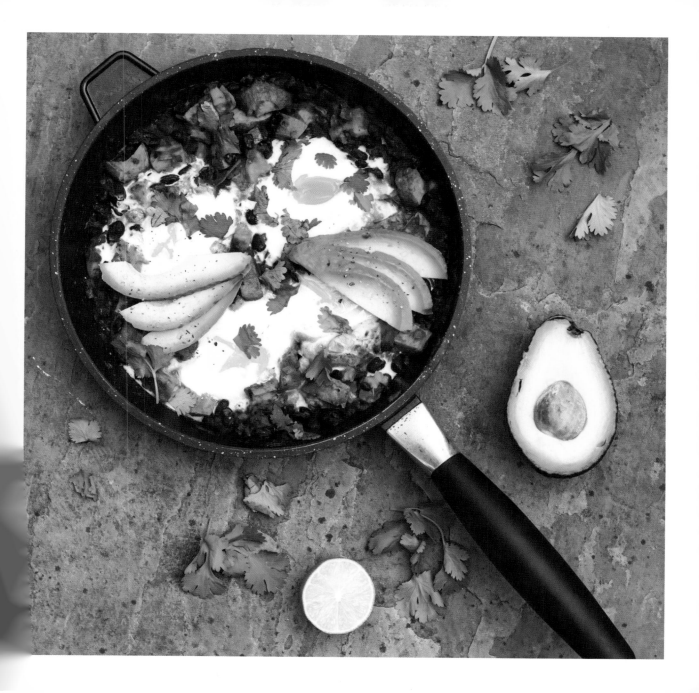

Superfoods

THE SUPERFOOD MYTH

Superfood (noun): *'a nutrient-rich food considered to be especially beneficial for health and wellbeing'*

Note: considered, not proven. The important distinction between marketing technique and science.

Despite the rise of the 'clean eating' movement that shuns processed foods and anything that isn't a 'whole food', we have also seen a rise in 'superfood' powders, which are definitely processed and not whole foods. Yet somehow we're led to believe that we need these for optimum health.

Extraordinary claims require extraordinary evidence, so let's examine the claims being made of various superfood powders and whether they stand up to the evidence. Specifically, baobab, maca, spirulina, wheatgrass and acai.

In 2007, marketing products as 'superfoods' became prohibited in the EU unless it is accompanied by a specific authorised health claim supported by evidence. Basically, instead of just calling anything a superfood, there now has to be some justification for it. Naturally, there are many ways people try to get around this, for example, calling things 'super greens' or 'super fruits'. This doesn't make the word superfood any more scientific, but at least it's not being thrown around as much as it used to be.

Taking high doses of vitamin C doesn't cure or prevent colds.

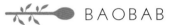 BAOBAB

Baobab powder is simply a powdered form of the fruit of the baobab tree, most commonly found in Africa. Baobab started out being recommended for thickening jam or as a sweetener for fruit-based drinks. It has since morphed into a superfood famous for being high in vitamin C. Sure, it has some fibre and antioxidants, but vitamin C is the big selling point.

Vitamin C is important in the body for skin, blood vessels, bones, cartilage and wound healing. Claims that it 'supports the immune system' are deliberately vague and don't mean anything. Basically, anything you eat effectively supports the immune system as it provides nutrients for the development of immune cells.

The reason the 'vitamin C cures colds' myth exists is thanks to Linus Pauling, the only person to receive two unshared Nobel Prizes and a good reminder that even the smartest people can fall for bullshit and pseudoscience.

Unfortunately, vitamin C doesn't cure colds. A review in 2013 concluded that regular ingestion of at least 200mg of vitamin C per day had absolutely no effect on the incidence of the common cold in the general population [1]. It also found that high dose vitamin C has no consistent or significant effect on duration or severity of symptoms. So the most you can hope for is that a three-day cold becomes shortened to merely around two days and nineteen hours, and that's if you're lucky. . . wow. It's a great placebo though! [2] Oops . . . just forget you read that part, I'm sure it'll still work.

While we're at it, it will almost definitely not cure cancer [3], sorry.

In conclusion, baobab powder is just a very expensive vitamin C powder, which most of the population don't need anyway because it's quite rare to become deficient. Don't bother.

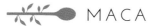 ## MACA

Maca is a Peruvian plant, the root of which looks like a turnip. It's this that gets turned into a powdered superfood, which can be either red, yellow or black.

Maca is supposedly an aphrodisiac, but research is still in early stages. It doesn't affect reproductive hormones in men [4], but it may improve sexual desire [5]. So does a placebo though, so who knows. It may also have a beneficial effect on sexual dysfunction in women [6], but as with men, this seems to be through affecting mood rather than sex hormones, although we don't know the supposed mechanism yet. It's also important to note that these studies are all quite small, and it's difficult to draw conclusions for seven billion people based on a sample size of around fifty.

Maca is also claimed to be a great pre- or post-workout tool as it supposedly increases energy. But at the time of writing, there were no studies I could find on maca and energy, or maca and muscle building in humans.

Finally, maca is supposed to be an 'adaptogen' – a substance that helps the body adapt to stress and restore homeostasis. There's a lot of nutribollocks surrounding this word, with vague notions of improving health, usually without a specified mechanism or explanation. (Note: please don't Google 'are adaptogens real?'; the amount of BS you'll come across is incredible.) As a result, maca has been promoted online as a treatment for menopausal symptoms. But again, as you may have guessed, there's no conclusive evidence [7].

I've seen products like this being hailed as having 'no downsides', which I would fundamentally disagree with. The safety of maca hasn't been proven yet. Encouraging people to swap their HRT for maca to treat menopausal symptoms despite the lack of evidence is not what I'd consider safe, and anecdotally I know of many young people who experienced side effects from just a teaspoon of the stuff. I wouldn't call that 'no downsides', even if only anecdotally.

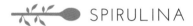 ## SPIRULINA

Spirulina is a cyanobacterium, or blue-green algae, otherwise known as pond scum. If that hasn't already put you off, maybe this next bit will.

Cyanobacteria can produce a neurotoxin called BMAA (a substance that is poisonous or destructive to nerve tissue). Right now, it's uncertain whether spirulina can produce BMAA (one study suggests no [8], while another says yes [9]). Not only that, but samples of spirulina have also been found to contain another neurotoxin called anatoxin-a, also known as Very Fast Death Factor or VFDF (don't tell me that scientists aren't good at naming things!) [10]. Great.

Spirulina is said to absorb heavy metals and toxins from the environment (see chapter 4 for a full take-down of detoxes), which is why there's a higher risk of contamination, as this absorption can occur before it's even harvested. Ironic for something that's supposed to detoxify you.

Spirulina is also hailed as a complete protein, meaning it features all nine essential amino acids. Considering a serving is one teaspoon (around 3g), even if it does contain 60–70% protein, that's still only around 2g of protein. Not really significant in the context of your overall diet.

So, on the upside, you'll get some protein in your diet from spirulina, but you'll also have potential exposure to neurotoxins and therefore higher risk of neurodegenerative diseases [11]. Thanks, I'll pass.

Oh, and did I mention that despite supplement companies claiming spirulina to be a good source of B12 (something lacking in vegan and sometimes vegetarian diets), spirulina actually contains pseudovitamin B12 [12], which is biologically inactive in humans and could even reduce the absorption of real B12? So please don't take spirulina as a B12 supplement, it won't help.

Overall, spirulina doesn't contain any nutrients that cannot be found in other foods at a reduced cost and easier availability. And it tastes absolutely vile. It gives everything it touches a dark green pond flavour. Why would you want to eat something that doesn't even taste good?

PIXIE TIP
Spirulina isn't a good source of B12, so please don't use it as a supplement.

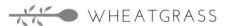 WHEATGRASS

I once gave my mother a wheatgrass shot. She gagged and almost threw up. I wish I had filmed it; it was hilarious.

Wheatgrass is simply the sprouts of the common wheat plant, which are either powdered or juiced. But don't panic; because it's harvested before the wheat seed grows, it's gluten free, which obviously means the wellness industry has instantly slapped a glowing halo of health on it.

Seriously though, wheatgrass is hailed as some kind of 'wonder plant' that has magical properties and infinitely more vitamins and minerals than other vegetables. 'Alkalising', 'detoxifying', 'immune-boosting'. . . these words mean absolutely nothing. They are nothing but bullshit marketing buzzwords to get you to buy something that offers no benefit over a head of broccoli.

One of the most bizarre claims about wheatgrass is that because it contains chlorophyll it helps 'oxygenate your blood'. I love claims like this because all I need to show how wrong it is, is a simple equation from GCSE biology. The equation for photosynthesis in plants (which is where chlorophyll comes from):

$$\text{CARBON DIOXIDE} + \text{WATER} + \text{LIGHT} \longrightarrow \text{GLUCOSE} + \text{OXYGEN}$$

Have you spotted it? Even if you did have chlorophyll molecules floating around in your blood, there's no way it can produce oxygen, because there's no light! Your blood vessels are inside your body, and if light is reaching your blood you should probably be more concerned that you might die. You oxygenate your blood by breathing in oxygen through your lungs, not by eating plants.

The other problem with this is that it implies your body can't tell the difference between haemoglobin and chlorophyll. Yes, they look similar, but the enzymes in your body are highly specific. Your body doesn't see chlorophyll and just decide 'that'll do, that's close enough'. This specificity is key to survival. Plus, chlorophyll is sensitive to extreme pH, so as soon as it hits your (highly acidic) stomach, it's digested just like everything else.

Along that same wavelength, wheatgrass contains plant enzymes, which are claimed to help with digestion. But enzymes are produced by organisms specifically for their own use, and so plant enzymes are subtly different to human enzymes. This means they get broken down as part of digestion just like any other protein would (remember all enzymes are proteins). Your body doesn't recruit enzymes from other organisms, they're highly specific.

Wheatgrass isn't uniquely special. It contains vitamins and minerals just like any other vegetable. It doesn't contain significantly larger amounts either. If you like the taste (seriously, how?), then go for it, it's not going to do any harm.

But if, like me, you find the taste or smell nauseating, you could eat literally any other green vegetable instead and still get the benefits.

 ## ACAI

Acai, aside from being constantly mispronounced (its: ah-SIGH-ee not ah-KAI), is an exotic berry with an apparently ridiculously high antioxidant score. It became famous as a weight loss tool on Oprah and the Dr Oz show in the US, despite having no evidence to support this claim (but hey, when has that ever stopped anyone).

But aren't antioxidants a good thing? They are indeed, but as with all things, only up to a point.

Everyone has heard of antioxidants, but I'm guessing few people know exactly how they work. Antioxidants protect you from cell damage and DNA damage that can lead to accelerated signs of ageing and, in some cases such as UV damage, can lead to cancer. This cell damage occurs because of oxidative stress – the process by which oxygen-based compounds, also known as reactive oxygen species (ROS), are made. ROS are highly reactive species and so want to react with whatever they can find, and quickly, even proteins, DNA or other cell components, thereby damaging them. ROS can occur simply as waste products from cell metabolism (as energy production requires oxygen) or from environmental stresses such as UV or heat exposure.

Some antioxidants are made by the body, such as superoxide dismutase, but they can also be found in food. Vitamins A, C and E, beta-carotene and polyphenols all have antioxidant capacity.

Based on all of this, you'd expect a greater consumption of antioxidants to be associated with better health and even lower cancer rates, right? We know that people with high consumption of fruit and vegetables have a lower incidence of cancer [13], but is that due to the carrot or the beta-carotene? The orange or the vitamin C? We also know that individuals with cancer have lower levels of beta-carotene in their blood [14], and that individuals with high levels of vitamin C in their blood have a reduced risk of stroke [15], but all we have here is correlation, it doesn't prove that one causes the other.

A logical next step would be to see if actively supplementing with antioxidants improves health. It doesn't. Supplementing with vitamin A, vitamin E or beta-carotene is associated with increased mortality [16], so you're actually more likely to die if you supplement with these than if you don't.

How can this possibly be the case? As always, too much of a good thing can be a bad thing. Free radicals, or ROS, aren't a human design flaw, they have a purpose. White blood cells use free radicals to help them kill bacteria, and if there is too much damage in a cell then free radicals signal for it to undergo apoptosis (programmed cell death). Too many antioxidants could allow damaged cells to survive for longer because it disrupts the cell signalling via free radicals, and damaged cells in your body is definitely not what you want.

PIXIE TIP
You can have too much of a good thing, and that also applies to antioxidants.

The idea that you need expensive powders in order to be healthy is ridiculous and elitist. You can't negate an unhealthy lifestyle simply by consuming a teaspoon of green powder. It doesn't work that way. There's also nothing in these powders that you can't get easily and more cheaply elsewhere

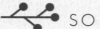 ## SO WHERE DOES THIS LEAVE US?

All these products have several things in common: they're exotic, expensive and have a mountain of dubious health claims to persuade you to part with money for them. And most of them taste pretty rubbish too. The idea that you need expensive powders in order to be healthy is ridiculous and elitist.

You can't negate an unhealthy lifestyle simply by consuming a teaspoon of green powder. It doesn't work that way. There's also nothing in these powders that you can't get easily and more cheaply elsewhere.

Baobab: If you're after vitamin C, there are so many easy ways to get vitamin C into your diet simply by eating certain fruits and vegetables like oranges, berries or peppers.

Maca: If you're after energy then coffee is your best friend. Coffee is not 'unhealthy', in fact it can actually reduce your risk of dying [17] (as well as helping you not to kill people around you first thing in the morning). A lack of energy could also be a sign that you need more fuel (i.e. food) or that you're deficient in certain micronutrients such as B12 or iron. Maca won't treat the underlying issue there.

Spirulina: If plant sources of protein are what you're after, then I can recommend a whole host of alternatives that give you way more protein per serving and don't taste like pond water. Although they aren't always complete proteins, by combining them properly you can ensure every dish will have a complete set of essential amino acids.

Wheatgrass: If you're after more greens, then you're better off eating any green vegetable instead. I guarantee they'll taste better.

Acai: Supplementing with antioxidants may not be the best idea, but getting them from fruits and vegetables means you'll get a whole host of other benefits without the potentially risky high levels of vitamins.

So you see, you simply don't need them, as the following recipes will show.

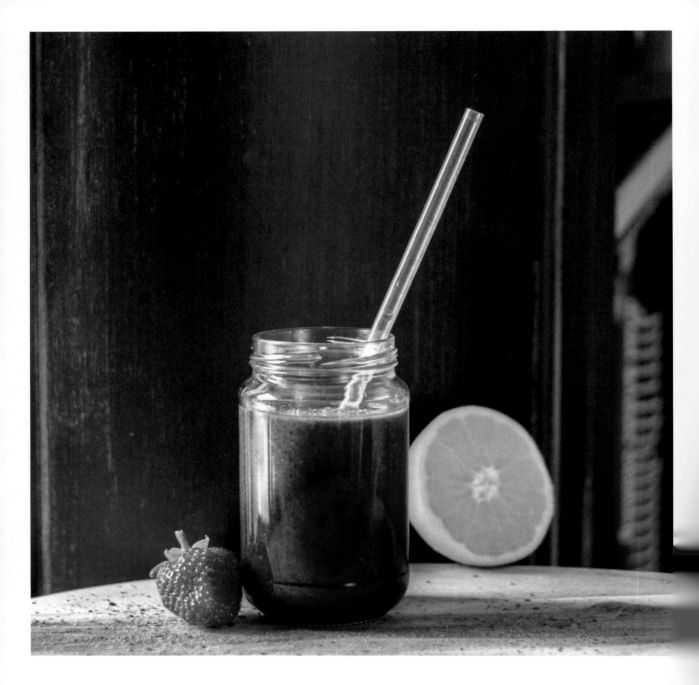

ORANGE & BERRY SMOOTHIE

SERVES 1

- 1 banana (around 70-100g)
- 80g frozen blueberries
- 80g frozen strawberries
- 1 orange, juice and pulp
- 1 tbsp ground flaxseed

Sure, baobab can give you some vitamin C, but a single orange can give you your entire recommended daily intake, whilst tasting a whole lot better too. In this recipe, I recommend adding the orange pulp as well as the juice to get some extra fibre in there.

Put all the ingredients into a blender in the order written.

Blitz until smooth, scraping the sides of the blender if you need to.

Pour into a tall glass to serve.

SUMMER ROLL SALAD WITH MANGO DRESSING

SERVES 2

- 200g rice noodles
- 1 red pepper, finely sliced
- 100g cucumber, finely sliced
- 100g carrot, finely sliced
- 100g beansprouts
- Small handful of fresh mint leaves, roughly chopped
- Small handful of fresh Thai basil or coriander leaves, roughly chopped
- 1 red chilli, deseeded and finely sliced

For the dressing
- 1 mango (around 200g), peeled and chopped
- 1 lime, juiced
- Pinch of chilli flakes
- 1 tbsp soy sauce
- Small handful of fresh Thai basil or coriander leaves

I first made my own spring rolls on a boat in Ha Long Bay. They were the fried kind rather than the fresh kind, though. Unfortunately, rice paper isn't always easy to find, so I've decided to take the ingredients that would normally go in rice paper rolls and turn them into a salad instead. The dressing really makes it, and thanks to the mango, it also has plenty of vitamin C, more so than a serving of baobab anyway.

Cover the rice noodles in hot water and set aside.

To make the dressing, put the mango flesh into a blender or food processor with the lime juice, a pinch of chilli flakes, soy sauce and Thai basil or coriander and blend until smooth.

Drain the water off the noodles and mix in 2 tablespoons of the dressing.

Mix in the vegetables and the herbs.

Drizzle over the remaining dressing and sprinkle with fresh chilli.

TIP Want more protein? Try adding salmon, prawns, chicken or tofu to your salad.

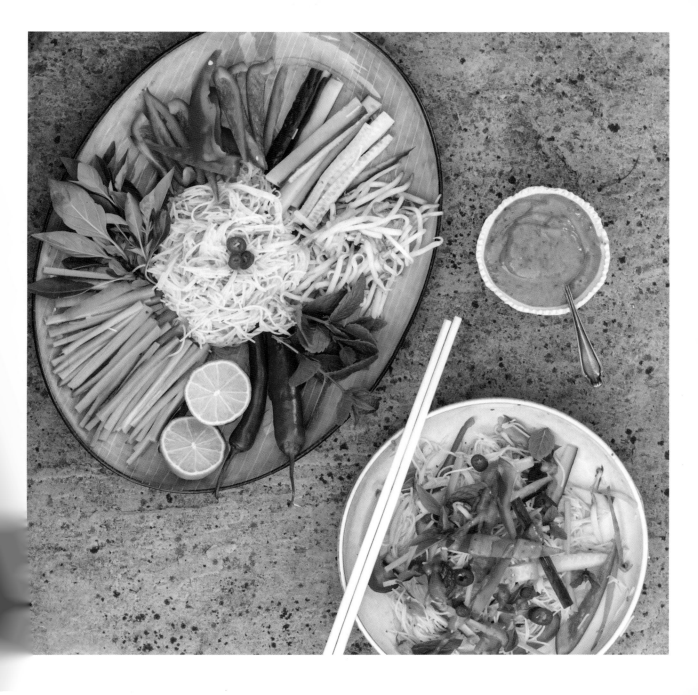

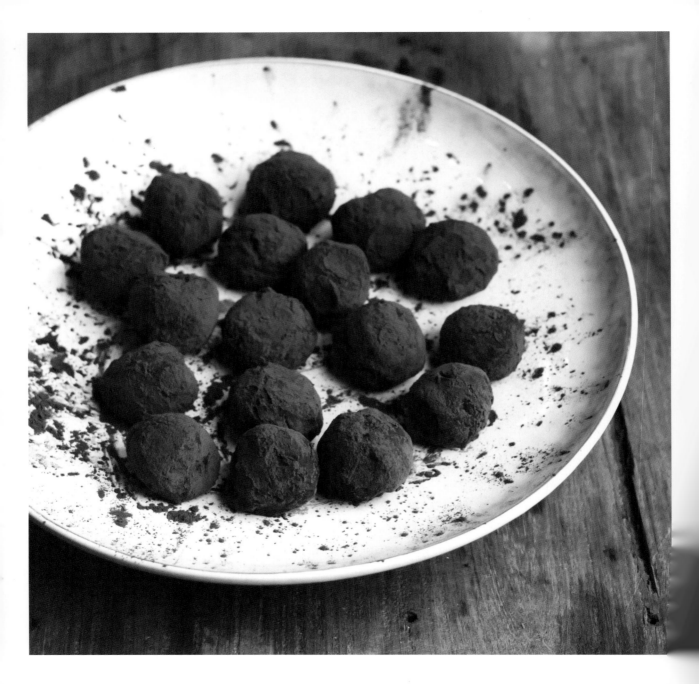

MOCHA TRUFFLES

MAKES AROUND 20

- 200g dark chocolate
- 240ml double cream
- 2 tsp stevia
- 1 tbsp instant coffee
- Cocoa powder for dusting

Not only does coffee work wonders at waking you up in the morning, it also tastes great when mixed with chocolate and in desserts, which is more than can be said for maca. In my experience, everything maca touches ends up tasting like freeze-dried clay, and not at all like the caramel it's supposed to. Coffee, on the other hand, just makes everything better.

Break the chocolate into a bowl.

Heat the cream and stevia in a saucepan, until the edges begin to bubble.

Pour the cream onto the chocolate and stir until the chocolate has melted and the mixture is smooth and silky.

Add the instant coffee and taste. Add more if you feel like it.

Leave the mixture to cool in the fridge for 1–2 hours.

Once cooled, roll into small 10p-sized balls and coat in cocoa powder.

Chill for another hour in the fridge or until ready to serve.

COFFEE SMOOTHIE

SERVES 1

- 1 banana (100g if you like bitter coffee or 150g if you like it sweeter)
- 200ml milk of your choice (I like oat milk)
- 1 tsp instant coffee granules
- Pinch of cinnamon

If you need waking up in the morning, I promise you this will work way better than maca. Because that's what coffee is supposed to do.

Blend the ingredients together in a blender or food processor.

Taste. If too bitter, add more banana.

Serve.

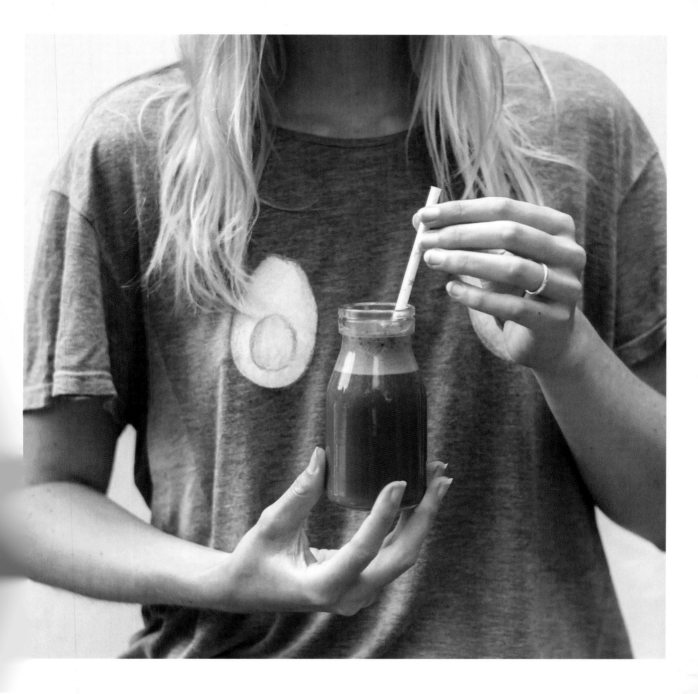

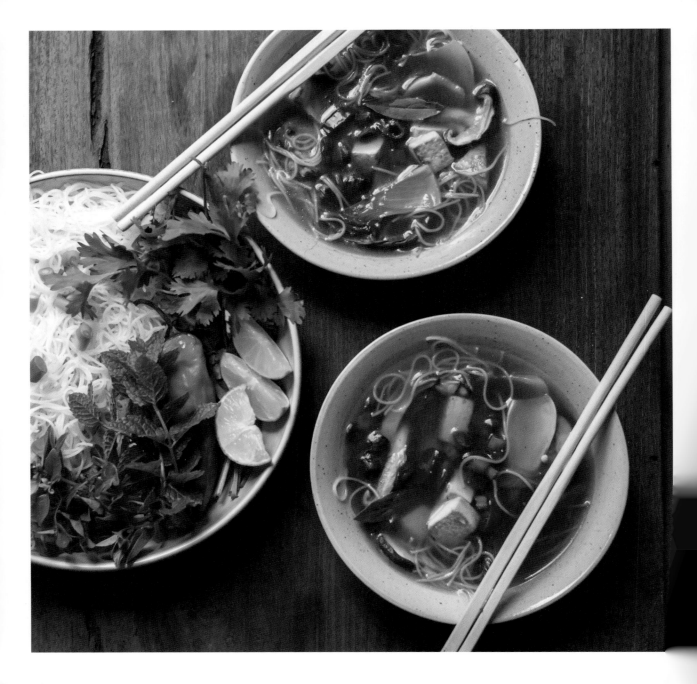

VEGGIE PHO

SERVES 2

- Stir-fry oil or sesame oil
- 2 star anise
- 1 cinnamon stick
- ½ tsp whole cloves
- 1 white onion (around 110g), peeled and quartered
- 1 x 2.5cm piece of fresh ginger
- 1 vegetable stock cube
- Plenty of soy sauce
- 125g shiitake mushrooms, sliced
- 150g tofu, cubed
- 100g pak choy
- 200g rice noodles
- Bunch of fresh herbs: coriander, Thai basil, mint
- 1 spring onion, chopped
- 1 red chilli, deseeded and sliced (optional)

I was taught to make pho by an old Vietnamese lady in a one-to-one cooking class in Hoi An. This isn't that exact recipe, but it's pretty similar. Plus it contains tofu, which is a complete protein like spirulina, while tasting a thousand times better. Even if you don't like tofu, it still tastes better, because nothing tastes as terrible as pond.

Heat a glug of oil in a saucepan over a medium heat, then add the star anise, cinnamon stick and cloves and fry for 2 minutes. Add the onion quarters to the pan along with the fresh ginger, vegetable stock cube, 1 tablespoon of the soy sauce and 1 litre of water. This will form your stock. Cook this gently for 30 minutes.

In the meantime, fry the mushrooms in a little oil and soy sauce until soft. Remove from the pan and set aside.

Fry the tofu in a little oil and soy sauce. Remove from the pan and set aside. Cut the base off the pak choy and separate the leaves. Strain the stock and pour it back into the saucepan. Add the pak choy and leave for 5 minutes. Season well with extra soy sauce or salt.

Cook the noodles according to the packet instructions.Divide the noodles between two bowls and put the herbs, spring onions and chilli (if using) into serving bowls. Add the mushrooms and tofu to the broth and ladle it over the noodles. Sprinkle your bowl with a mixture of herbs, spring onions and chilli if you like it hot.

VEGETABLE & CHICKPEA PAELLA

SERVES 4

- Olive oil
- 1 onion (around 110g), peeled and finely diced
- 2 garlic cloves
- 1 vegetable stock cube
- 200g paella rice
- 1 tbsp paprika
- 1 tsp saffron
- 150g portabellini mushrooms, sliced
- 1 red pepper, sliced
- 1 yellow pepper, sliced
- 100g tomatoes, diced
- Salt and pepper
- 1 x 400g tin of chickpeas, drained and rinsed
- Chopped fresh parsley leaves, to serve

Spirulina may be a complete protein, but so is this meal. Combining rice and beans means this meal has all the amino acids your body needs. Seeing as a serving of spirulina has around 3g of protein, and this meal definitely has more, you're much better off just eating this. Also, it doesn't taste like a pond, so it automatically wins.

Heat a glug of olive oil in a deep-sided frying pan over a medium heat. Add the diced onion and stir for 5 minutes.

Peel and crush the garlic, add it to the pan and stir for another few minutes.

Pour 500ml of boiling water over the stock cube and stir until dissolved. Add the rice to the pan and stir for a few minutes, then add the vegetable stock.

Add the spices, followed by the veggies and season with salt and pepper. Add more water if and when needed to stop the rice from drying out. Stir regularly to avoid sticking.

When the rice is almost ready, add the chickpeas. Taste and adjust the seasoning if necessary, particularly if more salt is needed.

Serve immediately with a sprinkling of fresh parsley.

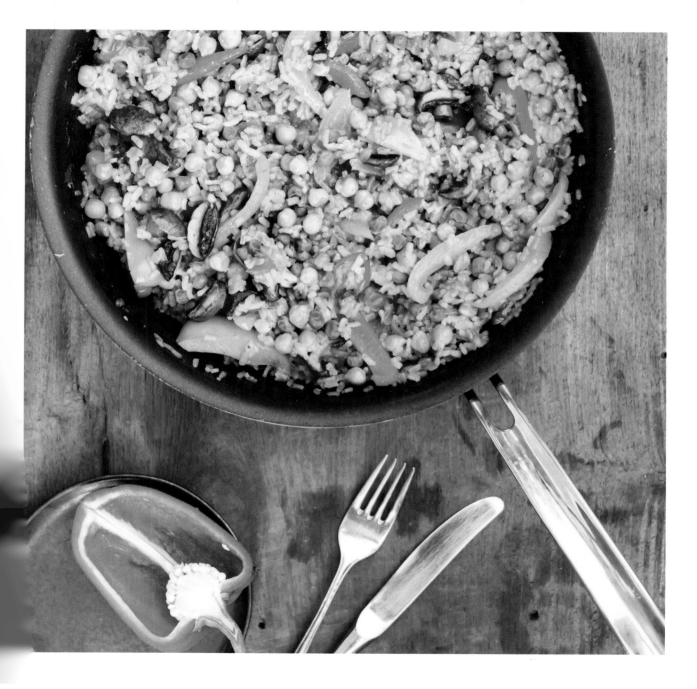

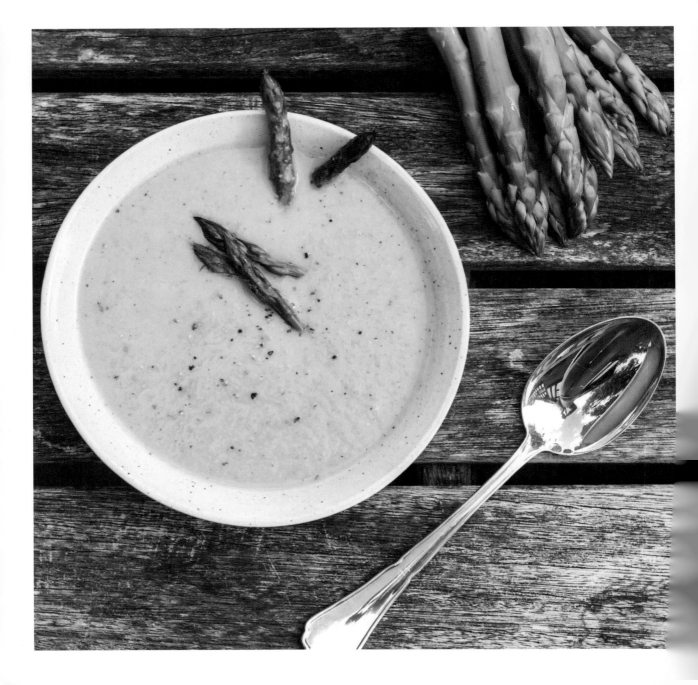

ASPARAGUS SOUP

SERVES 2

- Olive oil
- 3 garlic cloves
- 1 onion (around 110g), peeled and roughly chopped
- 500g asparagus
- 1 vegetable stock cube
- Salt and pepper
- 1-2 tbsp lemon juice

Asparagus tastes way better than wheatgrass. And asparagus soup tastes way better than wheatgrass soup. That's pretty much all you need to know!

Heat a glug of olive oil in a large saucepan over a medium heat.

Peel and crush the garlic and add it to the pan with the chopped onions. Fry for a couple of minutes.

Snap off the woody ends of the asparagus and cut the remaining part into thirds. Add these to the pan and stir for a couple of minutes.

Pour 700ml of boiling water over the stock cube and stir until completely dissolved. Add the stock to the pan and bring up to the boil.

Use a hand blender or food processor to transform the mixture into a deliciously creamy green soup. If the soup is not thick enough, return to the pan and allow it to cook down for a few more minutes over the heat.

Season with salt, pepper and lemon juice and serve with crusty bread.

GREENS & BEANS SALAD

SERVES 3-4

- 1 sweet potato (around 200g), peeled and cubed
- Olive oil
- Pinch of salt
- Pinch of paprika
- 250g asparagus
- 200g tenderstem broccoli
- 100g spinach leaves
- 1 large avocado, cubed
- 100g sugar snap peas
- 1 x 400g tin of chickpeas, drained and rinsed
- 1 x 400g tin of kidney beans, drained and rinsed
- 1 jar basil pesto (190g)

Wheatgrass tastes shit. Luckily green vegetables like broccoli, asparagus, sugar snap peas and spinach all taste great, especially all together. Conveniently, they all appear in this delicious salad that gives you six portions of vegetables (seven if you include the beans, and you should) all in one go.

Preheat the oven to 200°C fan/220°C conventional/gas mark 7.

Spread the sweet potato cubes over a baking tray, drizzle with olive oil and season with salt and paprika. Roast in the oven for around 20 minutes, until cooked through.

In the meantime, remove the woody ends from the asparagus and cut the stems into thirds.

Cut the broccoli in half. Steam or boil the broccoli for 5 minutes and the asparagus for 3-4 minutes, until slightly soft but still with some bite.

Slice large spinach leaves and cut the avocado into cubes.

Put everything into a bowl: cooked sweet potato, cooked greens, raw sugar snap peas, spinach, avocado, chickpeas and beans. Add the pesto and toss to coat.

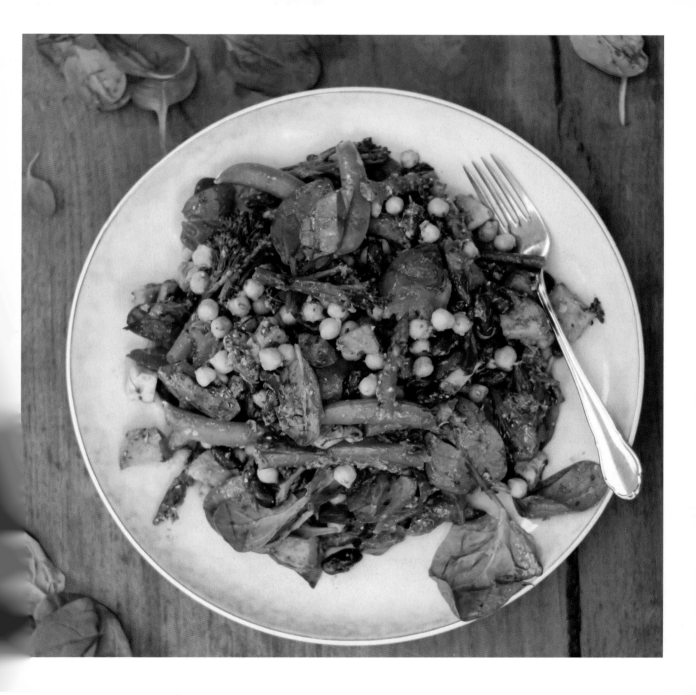

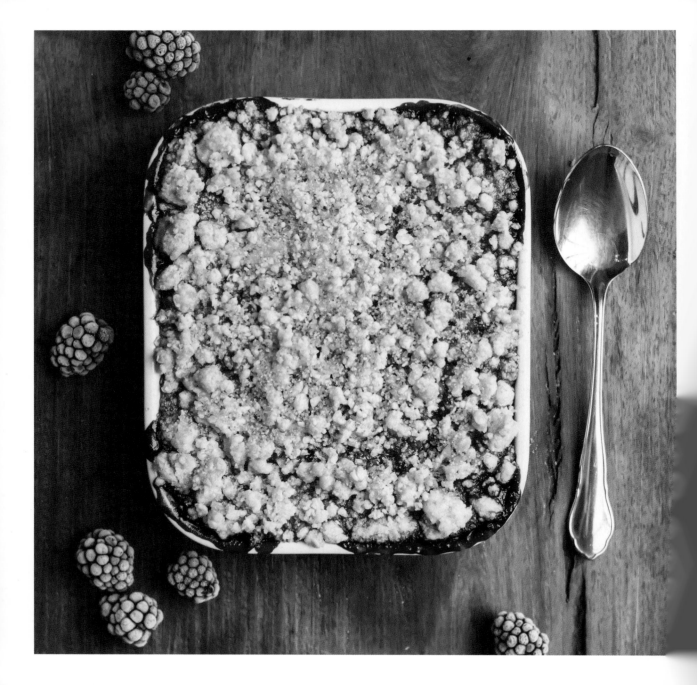

BERRY CRUMBLE

SERVES 4-6

- 150g blueberries
- 150g strawberries
- 150g blackberries
- 2 tbsp maple syrup
- 175g plain white flour
- 125g unsalted butter, softened not melted
- 125g Demerara sugar
- 1 tsp cinnamon
- 2 tbsp rolled oats or flaked almonds
- Custard, vanilla sauce or yoghurt, to serve

Blueberries, strawberries and blackberries are wonderful examples of British berries. Why do you need acai berries from the other side of the world when we have perfectly good ones here? And they taste brilliant in crumbles.

Preheat the oven to 150°C fan/170°C conventional/gas mark 3.

Heat the berries and maple syrup in a saucepan and cook down gently for 15 minutes.

In a bowl, mix together the flour and butter with your hands to form a crumb.

Mix in the sugar, cinnamon and oats, again with your hands.

Pour the fruit into the bottom of a casserole dish.

Gently pour the crumble on top. Try to distribute it evenly and once it's on, don't spread it around.

Bake for 30 minutes, until the top is crunchy and delicious. Serve with custard, vanilla sauce, or yoghurt.

TIP You can also use frozen berries for this crumble – just defrost them before cooking and get rid of any excess water.

NO-ACAI BOWL

SERVES 1

- 1 frozen sliced banana (around 100-120g)
- 80g frozen blueberries
- 80g frozen strawberries
- Splash of milk (any works)
- Awesome toppings: banana slices, berries, coconut flakes, granola, sprigs of fresh mint

Acai bowls can be very hit-and-miss. I've had some really icy, horrible ones and some delicious ones, which also tended to have a load of other delicious ingredients in it like frozen blueberries. This makes sense, because the acai we get here doesn't really taste like much, whereas blueberries do. So why not save yourself some money (and air miles) by just making an acai bowl without the acai – a no-acai bowl.

You're going to need a strong blender for this one. Add the ingredients to the blender in the order shown.

Add the milk in small amounts, as needed. Be patient with it and scrape the sides of the blender often. The final mixture should be smooth and super thick.

Pour this into a bowl and assemble the toppings. Go haphazard if you're in a rush or place carefully to showcase it for Instagram. I won't judge.

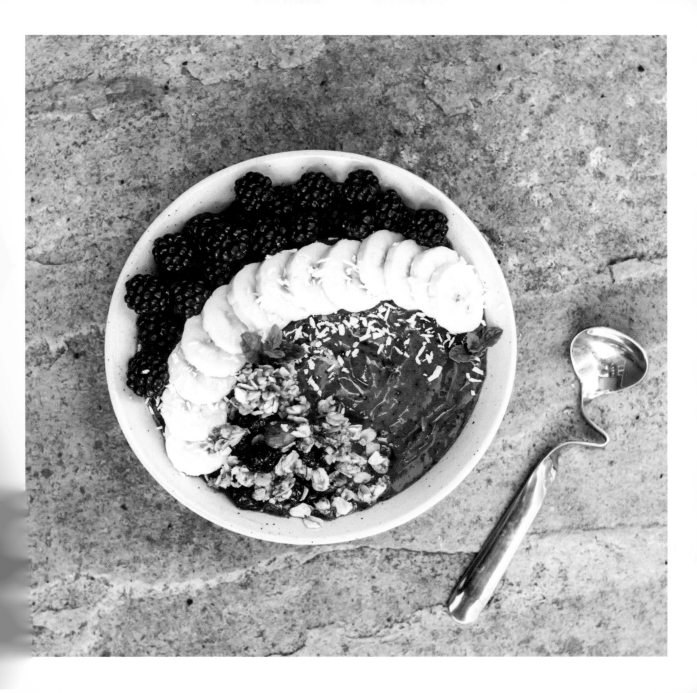

Alkaline

THE ALKALINE MYTH

Some myths are really hard to write about in a sensible manner, without resorting to intense snark and sarcasm. Not because I look down on the people who fall for diets like the alkaline diet (I mean I can't exactly talk), but because it makes me angry that there are those diet peddlers out there who would exploit people in this manner. Having said that, the alkaline diet is a subject that does bring my blood pressure up a few notches.

So what is the alkaline diet? The alkaline diet is based on the premise that the body functions best in a slightly alkaline state, and that illness is due to acidity in the body. Proponents of the alkaline diet say that what we eat and drink affects the pH of our bodies, including of the blood. So we need to eat an abundance of alkaline-forming foods (mainly fruits and vegetables), and avoid acid-forming foods (mainly meat and dairy). This is a whole load of nutribollocks that goes beyond just simply eating more vegetables.

ACID AND ALKALINE

pH is the measurement of hydrogen ion (H^+) concentration, which is a measure of acidity. pH measures how acidic or how alkaline a substance is. An acid has a low pH (or high concentration of hydrogen ions) and an alkali has a high pH. As a baseline, water at room temperature has a pH of 7, which is neutral.

Asking what's the pH of your body is like asking what the temperature of the Earth is: it varies! The saliva in your mouth has a neutral pH of 6 to 7.5, as this allows optimal function of salivary enzymes such as amylase (which breaks down carbohydrates). The stomach has a highly acidic pH of around 1.5–3, due to the presence of hydrochloric acid (HCl), and to ensure optimal functioning of enzymes to break down proteins. Once in the intestines, a substance called bile neutralises this acid to allow for the alkaline conditions needed for the enzymes in the small intestines. Finally, as the large intestines don't produce digestive enzymes the pH then goes back to being slightly acidic to neutral (5.5–7), finally resulting in excretion.

You don't have a 'body pH', the pH of your body varies from organ to organ.

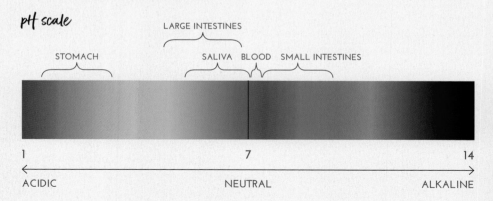

pH scale

LARGE INTESTINES

STOMACH SALIVA BLOOD SMALL INTESTINES

1 7 14

ACIDIC NEUTRAL ALKALINE

pH is tightly controlled, particularly the pH of the blood. Blood pH is between 7.35–7.45. Anything below pH 7.35 is considered acidosis, and anything above 7.45 is considered alkalosis. Blood pH is so tightly controlled because a deviation of more than 0.4 pH units either way is fatal. That means anything below pH 7 or above 7.7 is fatal.

The lungs, gut, kidneys and liver all play an important role in acid-base regulation. The body tries very hard to maintain pH within this 0.1 range, as the pH scale is a logarithmic scale, which means that a decrease of pH value by 1 unit (e.g. from 7 to 6) is equivalent to there being 10 times more hydrogen ions. That's big. Most enzymes function only within narrow pH ranges, and acid-base balance can affect electrolytes, hormones and bone synthesis. If the pH conditions of the cell change too much, the enzyme changes shape and denatures, rendering it useless. If it's unable to function, it won't be able to fulfil its role, whether that's food digestion, building hormones from scratch or deposition of bone material. The pH value needs to be maintained for proper functioning of every cell.

If you want to make yourself slightly more acidic then just hold your breath for 60 seconds. And if you want to make yourself slightly more alkaline then just hyperventilate. Neither feels particularly comfortable does it? You would be able to tell if your body was too acidic or alkaline. You can feel the difference. This works because the lungs respond quickly to pH changes by altering the amounts of carbon dioxide (CO_2) dissolved in the blood. This is the carbonate buffer system.

Ok hold up, what's a buffer system? I'm aware as we delve into the biochemistry some people will switch off; that's fine, just skip past this next section. For some of you though, me saying the body has extremely tight regulations called buffer systems to maintain pH is just not going to be enough. To sate your curiosity, take a deep breath, and read on for the science.

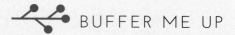 BUFFER ME UP

Buffers work by consuming small amounts of acid or alkali. There are three main buffering systems in the body:

1.   Protein buffer system
2.   Bicarbonate buffer system
3.   Phosphate buffer system

They all work in similar ways. Small amounts of extra acid or alkali are easily mopped up by proteins in the blood, including haemoglobin. The same goes for phosphate, but phosphate buffers only play a minor role as they're found in very low concentrations in the blood. The bicarbonate buffer system is the more interesting one.

The bicarbonate buffer system relies on the fact that all cells produce carbon dioxide as a waste product of metabolism (i.e. glucose + oxygen > water + carbon dioxide + energy). This carbon dioxide is released into the blood, and affects the pH as carbon dioxide is acidic. In the blood, carbon dioxide (CO_2) reacts with water (H_2O) to form a bicarbonate ion (HCO_3^-) and a hydrogen ion (H^+, an acid).

Cells can change their pH, as cells can change their metabolic rate, thereby changing the amount of carbon dioxide that they release into the blood. The lungs, however, are the main regulators of pH, as they allow you to breathe out the carbon dioxide to get rid of it. Changes in breathing rate affect carbon dioxide levels in the blood, hence why hyperventilation creates a more alkaline environment and hypoventilation (holding your breath) a more acidic environment. This is the main limitation of buffer systems: they are only a temporary solution and don't eliminate acid from the body. That's where your lungs and kidneys come in, by breathing out carbon dioxide and excreting

HCO_3^- (bicarbonate ions) via the urine.

I'm not telling you all this information to overwhelm you (although I'm aware it might be too late for that); what I want to get across is that pH regulation in your body is a highly intricate and complex process. So rather than just telling you that, I wanted to show you, to prove to you that this is the case. Your body has very precise mechanisms for detecting changes in pH, the same way it does for blood pressure, temperature and so on. This regulation is part of homeostasis (i.e. maintaining a constant internal environment).

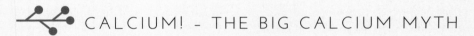 ## CALCIUM! – THE BIG CALCIUM MYTH

Interestingly, calcium can also act as a buffer to acid, which is why you'll hear people say that calcium counters the acid in meat, which leads to calcium loss from bones. In fact, there is no conclusive evidence to suggest that animal protein consumption is detrimental to bone health [1, 2, 3]. So how can this be? It seems that excess protein consumption actually increases calcium absorption in your body [4], and the calcium from the food is what ends up in the urine, not the calcium from your bones. So, yes, you lose more calcium in your urine, but it pretty much all comes from your diet rather than your skeleton. Your body is not using calcium from bones to neutralise the 'acidic load' of animal protein. Nope. Not unless you're not getting enough calcium from your diet, but conveniently calcium is found in dairy.

But wait! Isn't there a graph that shows countries with increased dairy consumption also have increased rates of osteoporosis? True, this graph exists. But firstly this is just a correlation and doesn't tell us which one causes the other. Secondly there are so many confounding variables there, such as overall

Contrary to popular 'health blogger' folklore, dairy doesn't actually leach calcium from your bones.

diet, specific other components of the diet such as vegetable consumption, and lifestyle factors such as stress.

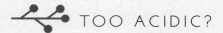 ## TOO ACIDIC?

The body produces more acids than alkalis, from food, food metabolism and production of carbon dioxide from respiration. Perhaps this is partly why the alkaline diet focuses on acidosis.

Symptoms of acidosis include weakness, disorientation and decrease in functioning of the central nervous system. In severe cases, it leads to coma and death.

Symptoms of alkalosis include over-excitability of the central and peripheral nervous systems, numbness and light-headedness (like what a panic attack feels like). In severe cases, it can lead to muscle spasms, convulsions, loss of consciousness and death.

Being 'too acidic' isn't something you can just quickly change by eating some greens; it involves hospitalisation and treatment with intravenous lactate. Being too alkaline is just as serious a problem, with treatment involving intravenous chloride solution. When you consume foods the pH of the food is changed in different parts of the body to match the ideal conditions of digestive enzymes: first acidic in the stomach then more alkaline in the intestines. No food can compete with the army of enzymes and their pH demands.

WHAT'S THE HARM?

From a purely nutritional perspective, the alkaline diet has some benefits, particularly as it encourages increased consumption of fruits and vegetables, something the general population definitely need more of – 70% of UK adults don't get their five a day [5].

So what's the harm? Surely adding more fruits and vegetables into your diet is a good thing, right? It is, but the problem comes when that good message gets buried in a deep steaming pile of (highly acidic) bullshit.

Here's what proponents of the alkaline diet have to say about it:

'People who remain too acid often display symptoms such as anxiety, diarrhoea, dilated pupils, extroverted behaviour, fatigue in early morning, headaches, hyperactivity, hypersexuality, insomnia, nervousness, rapid heartbeat, restless legs, shortness of breath, strong appetite, high blood pressure, warm dry hands and feet.'

To quote the 'Queen of Green' herself, Natasha Corrett, 'There are certain foods that are acid-forming . . . if you eat a lot of these foods your body has to work overtime and draw from the minerals in your bones to bring itself back to an alkaline state.'

The alkaline diet works, in the sense that it can be an effective weight loss tool. Given a set of simple rules to follow – 'good' and 'bad' foods become 'alkaline' and 'acidic' foods – and a calorie deficit, of course weight loss is a potential outcome. But apparently weight loss claims are not enough. Health claims vary from the relatively benign weight management and reduced acne to cancer. Yes, they went there. They claim to be able to cure cancer. This is where it gets messed up.

The alkaline diet theory states that the body functions optimally in an alkaline environment, and proponents vary in the direction of causation of acidity. Some say an acidic body is the root cause of all disease, whereas others simply say, 'disease cannot survive in an alkaline state and yet thrives in an acidic environment'. Or as Natasha Corrett says, 'The body can't get cancer in an alkaline state; cancer creates disease in the body through acidity.'

Cancer cells divide very quickly, and as a result they have huge energy demands. They use a form of energy production which doesn't require as much oxygen and produces lactate – which is acidic. It occurs in the microenvironment of cancer cells in some cases – but not all – and is not something that occurs in the whole body to make it acidic. This is a result of cancer, not the cause, and is also completely separate to blood pH.

If the key to health really is an 'alkaline state', then why the need to buy expensive machines that alkalise water, which is something they advocate? Why not just take some (highly alkaline) antacids instead? Because it doesn't work that way. If antacids prevented cancer then every person who's ever had heartburn would be immune.

It's true, an alkaline environment does kill cancer cells, but it also kills pretty much every other cell in the body too. Your cancer would be gone, but so would you.

Acidosis is a symptom not a cause of cancer. It can happen in response to cancer, severe diarrhoea, diabetes or liver failure to give a few examples. Acidosis doesn't cause these issues, and so eating alkaline doesn't treat the root cause, despite this being the apparent selling point.

But Natasha Corrett says eating acidic foods puts a strain on the body to maintain homeostasis, which can have long-term consequences. Well, wouldn't the same happen with eating only alkaline foods? Don't forget, blood pH is almost neutral. Would that not mean eating too alkaline would be putting a strain on the body, too? You can't just have it one way. Also, why does no one make this kind of argument for something like temperature which is also tightly regulated? Is constantly living at a temperature colder than our body temperature (37°C) also 'putting strain on our body'? No, we deal with it.

 ## WHY HAS IT BECOME POPULAR?

The alkaline diet has simple rules. It divides food into two simple categories, and says eat these but not these. It's a simple narrative. However, food rules like these can foster negative relationships with food, disrupt social lives and even lead to vitamin deficiencies.

The likes of Natasha Corrett claim that an acidic diet leaves you more likely to develop colds, bad skin and dull hair. If the shininess of your hair (which, by the way, is not guaranteed) is more important to you than your psychological wellbeing, then be my guest.

The alkaline diet plays on the fact that most people would have heard of pH and be vaguely familiar with it from GCSE chemistry, which immediately makes people think it's rooted in science, even though it's not. The very fact that lemons are seen as 'alkalising' should tell you just how inconsistent and unscientific the alkaline diet is. Lemon juice contains a decent amount of citric acid, yes acid, which is used as a preservative because it is an acid. Yet somehow this acid with a pH of around 2.2 magically becomes alkaline when you eat it? I don't think so.

Alkaline advocates even give you a 'sciencey' way of measuring the effectiveness of the diet by getting you to measure your urine pH (i.e. peeing on a stick). Conveniently you can usually buy these sticks on the websites of people claiming the effectiveness of the alkaline diet, along with expensive machines that alkalise your water. Unfortunately, these sticks won't tell you much about the pH of your body, as urine is a waste product and is external to your body, even when inside your bladder.

PIXIE TIP
Rather than focusing on the rigid rules of the alkaline diet, why not instead focus on getting enough fruit and vegetables into your diet?

Checking the pH of your urine is pretty harmless (although arguably a bit obsessive), but cancer is a whole other ball game. I believe there is a special circle of hell reserved for those who exploit vulnerable individuals such as those diagnosed with cancer. To give someone false hope like that and then blame them when it doesn't work out is inhuman. I would never blame someone for falling for false cancer cures, never. Having fallen for pseudoscience myself, of course I can understand how someone would be willing to try anything. But to exploit those people? Even if they believe in their 'treatment' fully and absolutely, would their patients dying on them not at least make them question whether they can do more? Do better? Change their practice?

Claiming that a treatment will treat or cure cancer without solid evidence is illegal in the UK under the Cancer Act 1939, which is why websites promoting the alkaline diet tend to have a robust disclaimer that the information they provide isn't intended to diagnose or cure. Why don't they provide this evidence? 'There is no scientific literature establishing the benefit of an alkaline diet for the prevention of cancer.' [6] So why not do studies and show the world how effective their treatment is? Is it because they're too scared deep down that it doesn't work, because all the research to date shows the alkaline diet is total nutribollocks [1, 2, 3]? It genuinely baffles, saddens and angers me more than anything else I've come across.

It comes down to this: a diet high in 'acidic' foods, that is, a diet low in fruits and vegetables, is a typical Western-type diet. We know this kind of diet has negative health consequences, but this is not because it makes your body 'acidic' in any way [7]. But if only eating acidic foods is bad then the same should apply to only eating alkaline foods. The logical conclusion is ditch the labels and dichotomy and just eat a balanced diet. Great, glad we cleared that up.

Checking the pH of your urine is pretty harmless, but cancer is a whole other ball game.

Many of the foods considered to be 'acidic' – such as most grains, beans, nuts, oils and cheese – have wonderful health benefits attached to them, not to mention they can transform the flavour of a dish and make it taste incredible. Hopefully, I've achieved that with this next set of recipes, and shown you that just because some of the ingredients are deemed to be 'acidic' doesn't mean you need to avoid them.

PIXIE TIP
Don't stress about the pH of your food, many wonderfully nutritious foods such as beans and grains, are considered 'acidic'!

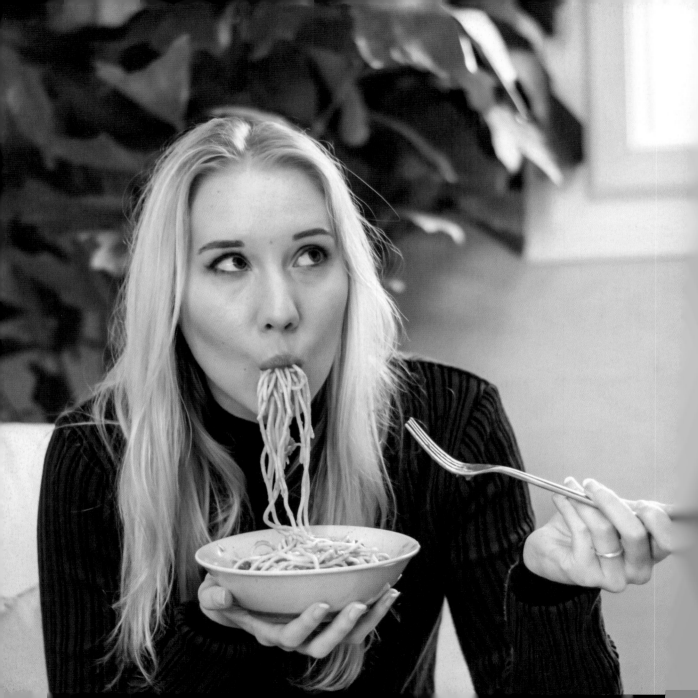

The alkaline diet plays on the fact that most people would have heard of pH and be vaguely familiar with it from GCSE chemistry, which immediately makes people think it's rooted in science, even though it's not

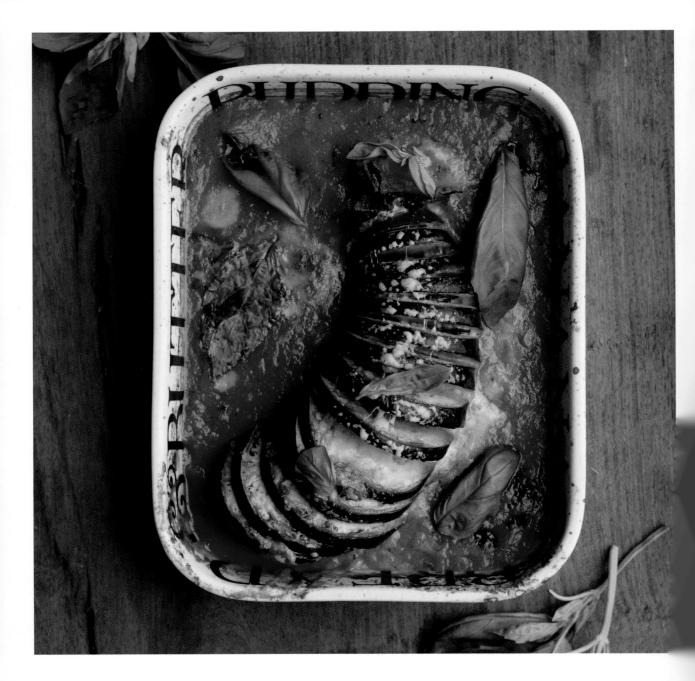

AUBERGINE PARMIGIANA

SERVES 2

- Olive oil
- 1 small onion (around 80-100g), peeled and roughly chopped
- 3 garlic cloves, peeled and crushed
- 1 x 400g tin of chopped tomatoes
- 1 tbsp tomato purée
- Salt and pepper
- Small bunch of fresh basil leaves, roughly chopped, plus extra for serving
- 1 aubergine (around 300g)
- 1 mozzarella ball (220g undrained weight)
- Finely grated Parmesan (as much as you want!)
- 20g fresh or dried breadcrumbs (optional)

This is a really delicious and impressive-looking veggie centrepiece. Sure, it has 'acidic' cheese but now you know that cheese doesn't actually leach calcium from your bones that shouldn't be a problem.

Preheat your oven to 180°C fan/200°C conventional/gas mark 6.

In a small saucepan, heat a little olive oil over a medium heat, then add the onion and fry for at least 5 minutes. Add the garlic and cook for another 5 minutes. Add the chopped tomatoes and the tomato purée. Allow to cook down for around 5 minutes, then season to taste with salt, pepper and a little basil. For a smooth sauce, blend to an even consistency. Or, if you prefer, you can leave it chunky.

Slice the aubergine almost all the way through but not quite so it's still all in one piece. Slice the mozzarella into thin slices. Pour the tomato sauce into the bottom of a large casserole dish

Place a piece of basil and a slice of mozzarella in between each aubergine segment. Put the aubergine on top of the tomato sauce. Sprinkle with a little Parmesan and the breadcrumbs (if using), and drizzle with olive oil. Cover with foil and place in the oven for 1 hour.

Remove the foil and add a generous amount of Parmesan. Put the dish back into the oven without the foil for another 10-15 minutes.

When ready, sprinkle a few more basil leaves on top and serve.

BLACK BEAN CHILLI

SERVES 3

- Olive or vegetable oil
- 1 onion (around 110g), peeled and finely diced
- 2 garlic cloves
- 1 tbsp paprika
- 1 tsp cumin
- Sprinkling of chilli flakes, to taste
- 1 x 400g tin of chopped tomatoes
- 1 vegetable stock cube
- 1 x 400g tin of black beans, drained and rinsed
- 1 x 400g tin of kidney beans, drained and rinsed
- Salt and pepper
- Plain yoghurt and fresh coriander, to serve

Did you know that beans are considered to be an 'acidic' food and therefore 'bad'? Doesn't make sense really considering they're such a wonderful source of protein and fibre. Ah well, at least they're combined here with nicely 'alkaline' onions and tomatoes, so I guess that balances it out? Oh wait, it doesn't matter, because the alkaline diet is bollocks. Phew.

Heat a little oil in a saucepan over a medium heat. Add the onion and cook for about 5 minutes.

Peel and crush the garlic and add to the onions. Stir for 2 minutes.

Add the paprika, cumin and chilli flakes. Stir for another minute.

Add the chopped tomatoes, then half fill the tin with water and add that too. Turn up the heat, and stir in the stock cube.

After 5 minutes, drain and rinse the beans, and add them to the pan.

Allow the chilli to cook down until much thicker, about 15–20 minutes.

Season with salt and pepper.

Serve with yoghurt and fresh coriander.

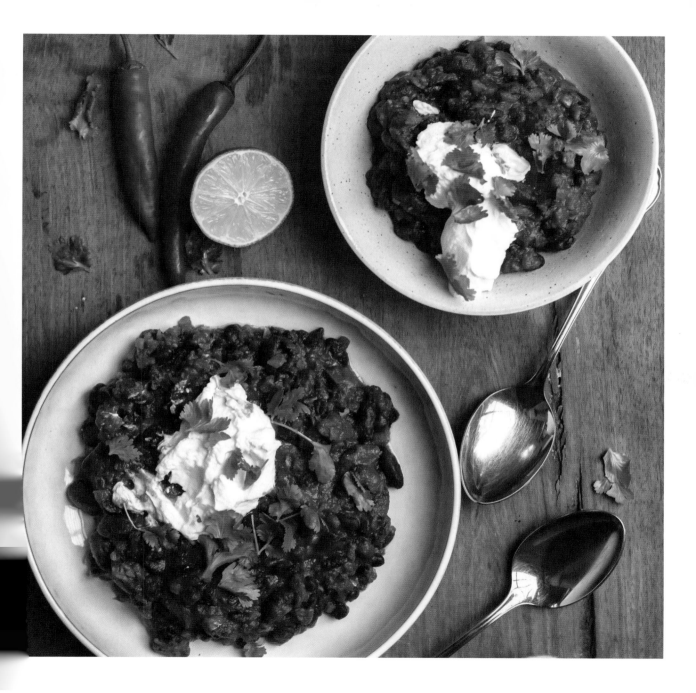

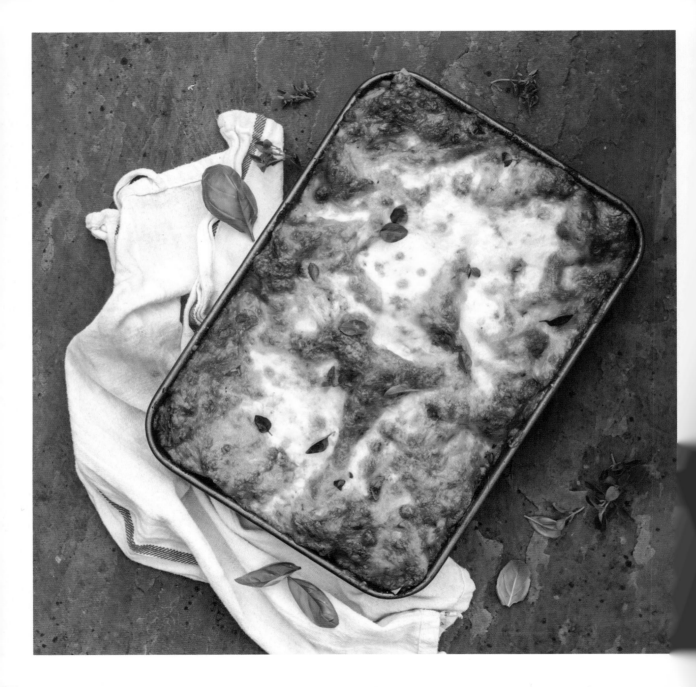

BUTTERNUT SQUASH LASAGNE

SERVES 6-8

- 1.4kg butternut squash
- Olive oil
- Salt and pepper
- 400g courgettes
- 1 onion (around 110g), peeled and finely diced
- 2 garlic cloves
- 680g passata
- 1 tbsp mixed herbs
- 1 tbsp chopped fresh basil
- 500ml crème fraîche
- 200g grated Parmesan
- 500g dried lasagne sheets
- 4 x 125g mozzarella balls, sliced

You will need
- A deep-sided ovenproof dish measuring approximately 23x33cm

Lasagne with vegetables instead of meat, surely that has to earn me some 'alkaline' points? Except for the fact that I've added a shitload of 'acidic' cheese, because, in my opinion, a lasagne without cheese just isn't worth having.

Preheat the oven to 200°C fan/220°C conventional/gas mark 7.

Peel the squash and slice into 5mm thick rings. Place on a lined baking tray, brush both sides with oil and season with salt and pepper. Roast in the oven for 30 minutes, then set aside to cool.

Thinly slice the courgettes lengthways, brush with olive oil and season with salt and pepper. Cook on both sides in a hot griddle pan or in the oven for a couple of minutes until cooked. Put to one side to cool.

To make the tomato sauce, heat a glug of olive oil in a small saucepan over a medium heat, add the diced onion and cook for 5 minutes.

Peel and crush the garlic and add to the pan, stirring for another 2 minutes.

Add the passata and herbs, and simmer for 15–20 minutes. >

BUTTERNUT SQUASH LASAGNE cont.

To make the white sauce, mix together the crème fraîche and 50g of the Parmesan, then season well with salt and pepper.

Lightly grease your dish with a little oil.

Time to layer up! Make sure to use quite thin layers of sauce so you have enough for all the layers. Start with a layer of lasagne sheets, followed by a thin layer of tomato sauce, some of the butternut squash, a thin layer of white sauce and a sprinkle of Parmesan, followed by more lasagne sheets, white sauce, courgette, more white sauce and more Parmesan and repeat the whole pattern. After the last lasagne sheets, finish with any of the remaining tomato sauce, a thick layer of mozzarella slices and the last of the Parmesan.

Turn the oven down to 170°C fan/190°C conventional/gas mark 5. Bake the lasagne for around 45 minutes, until golden brown and a knife slides through the lasagne sheets easily. Serve hot!

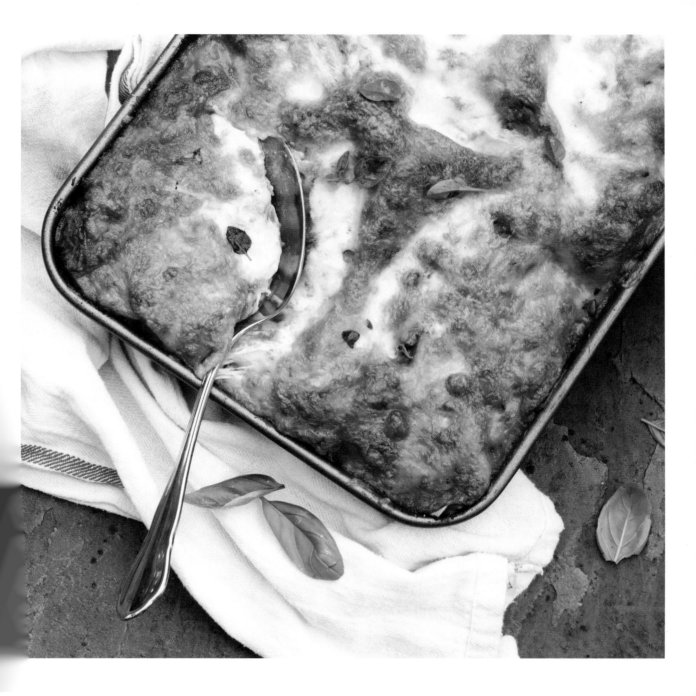

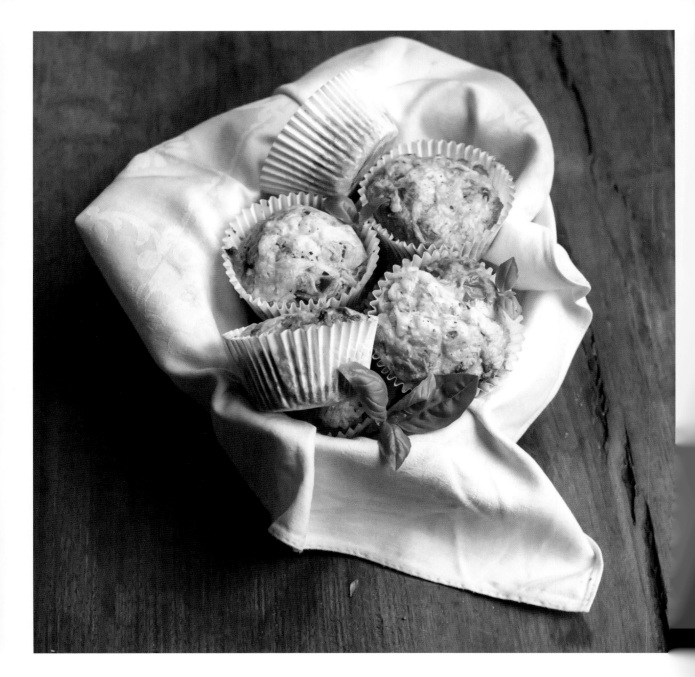

CHEESY MUFFINS

MAKES 9

- 200g wholemeal self-raising flour
- 100g courgette, grated and excess water removed
- 100g grated cheddar cheese, plus extra for sprinkling on top
- 100g cherry tomatoes, quartered
- 1 medium egg, beaten
- 50ml olive oil
- 150ml milk (any kind)
- 1 tsp paprika
- Salt and pepper

When something as basic as wheat flour is considered 'acidic' you know the alkaline diet really is a load of rubbish and just a disguised weight-loss diet. Eating these cheesy muffins won't make your body 'acidic'. Promise.

Preheat the oven to 200°C fan/220°C conventional/gas mark 7.

Mix all the ingredients together in a large bowl until fully incorporated and season with salt and pepper.

Fill nine muffin cases with equal amounts of the mixture.

Sprinkle some extra grated cheese on top of each one.

Place in the oven to bake for 15–20 minutes, until golden brown and an inserted toothpick comes out clean.

FALAFEL THREE WAYS

MAKES 8 FALAFEL

- Olive oil
- 1 small onion (around 80-100g), peeled and finely diced
- 1 x 400g tin of chickpeas, drained and rinsed
- 1 garlic clove
- 1 tbsp lemon juice
- 1 tbsp lemon zest
- 1 tsp ground cumin
- 1 tsp ground coriander
- 1 tsp mixed herbs
- 2 tbsp plain or wholemeal flour
- Salt and pepper

Variations

- Pink - add 150g cooked beetroot + 20g fresh breadcrumbs
- Green - add 10g fresh mint, parsley and basil
- Orange - add 200g cooked sweet potato, skin removed. Omit the flour

Not one, not two, but three kinds of falafel! So this is more like three recipes in one. Pick the one that sounds most appealing, or make all three and choose your favourite. Chickpeas are 'acidic'?! Oh come on, really? Screw this alkaline bollocks, and screw anyone who tells you that you can't eat falafel, you don't need that kind of negativity in your life.

Preheat the oven to 180°C fan/200°C conventional/gas mark 6.

Heat a little oil in a frying pan and cook the diced onions until soft.

Put the onions and into a food processor and add the remaining ingredients. Blitz until fully incorporated and smooth.

Form into 8 equal-sized balls and place on a baking tray lined with baking paper.

Place in the oven to bake for 15 minutes.

Remove the falafels from the oven and shallow fry in olive oil for a few minutes each side, until golden brown all over.

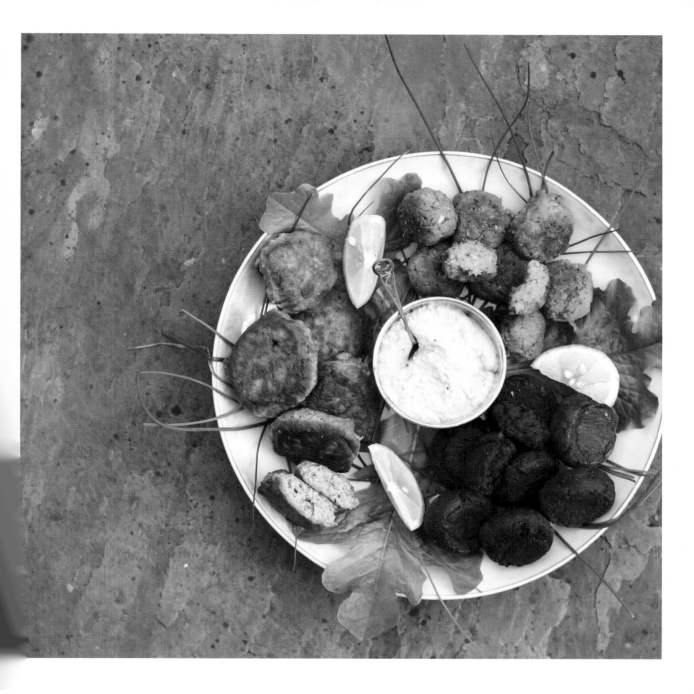

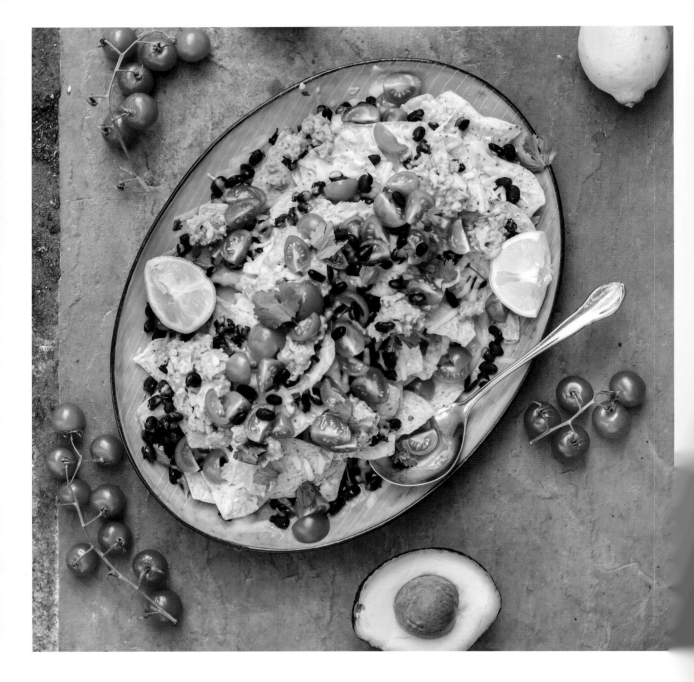

FULLY LOADED NACHOS

SERVES 4

- 200g salted tortilla chips
- 120g cheddar cheese, grated
- 1 x 400g tin of black beans, drained and rinsed
- 150g cherry tomatoes
- 2 tbsp lemon juice, plus wedges to serve
- Salt and pepper
- 1 large avocado (around 250g whole)
- Small handful of fresh coriander leaves (optional)

Corn is 'alkaline'! Rejoice and eat nachos to your heart's content. The acidic-yet-somehow-magically-alkaline lemon also makes an appearance.

Preheat the oven to 150°C fan/170°C conventional/gas mark 3.

In a shallow ovenproof dish or large plate, assemble a layer of tortilla chips with cheese and beans, then a second layer on top.

Bake in the oven until the cheese has melted.

In the meantime, make the salsa: finely dice the tomatoes and place in a small bowl with 1 tablespoon lemon juice and a pinch of salt.

To make the guacamole, mash the avocado in a small bowl with 1 tablespoon lemon juice and a pinch of salt and pepper.

When the cheese has melted, about 10 minutes, take the tortilla chips out of the oven, and dollop on the guacamole and salsa. Finish off with a sprinkling of fresh coriander leaves (if using) and serve with lemon wedges.

LENTIL & SWEET POTATO BURGERS

MAKES 4

- 100g red split lentils
- 150g sweet potato, peeled and chopped into 1-cm cubes
- 1 small onion (around 80g), peeled and very finely diced
- 1 garlic clove
- 1 tsp ground cumin
- 1 tsp paprika
- 1 tsp ground coriander
- Salt and pepper
- 10g fresh breadcrumbs
- 1 medium egg, beaten
- Olive oil
- Flour, for dusting
- Lettuce leaves, tomato slices, avocado and/or hummus, to serve

Combine 'acidic' lentils and 'alkaline' sweet potato and what do you get? A seriously delicious burger, that's what.

Cook the lentils in a pan of boiling salted water for 7 minutes then drain of all excess water.

Put the sweet potato in a mixing bowl and microwave for 5 minutes until soft. Mash roughly, then add the onion, garlic, lentils and spices. Season with salt and pepper then mix well and taste to check the seasoning. Mix in the breadcrumbs and egg.

Divide the mixture into four and form into burgers around 2–3cm thick. If the mixture is too dry to sork with, add a little oil. If it's too wet add a few more breadcrumbs or a little flour. Dusting your hands with flour can help with the shaping process, too.

Heat a frying pan over a medium heat, and add around 1 tablespoon of olive oil. When hot, place one burger gently in the frying pan and press down slightly with a spatula. Fry on both sides for a couple of minutes until slightly brown. Make sure to flip very carefully and no more than once to help them hold their shape. Add more olive oil each time you fry another burger. I recommend cooking them one at a time as they can be more delicate than meat-based burgers.

Serve in buns with lettuce, tomato, avocado and/or hummus.

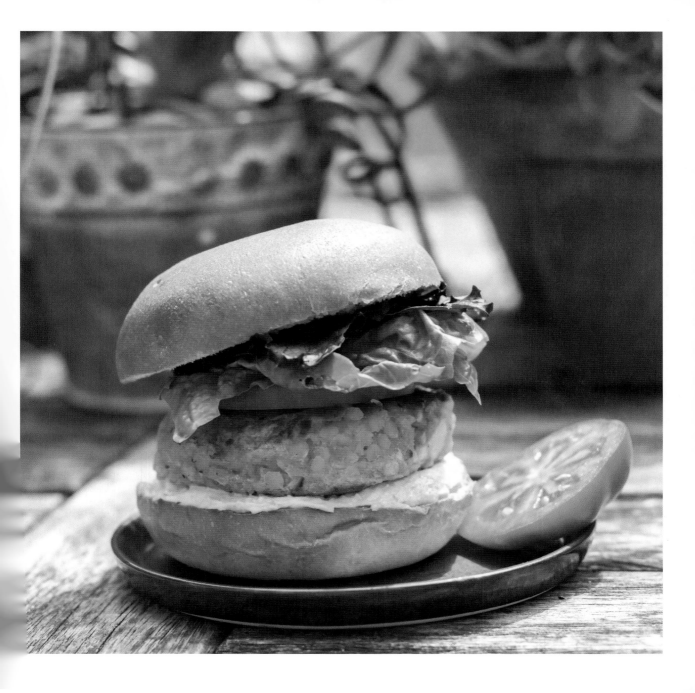

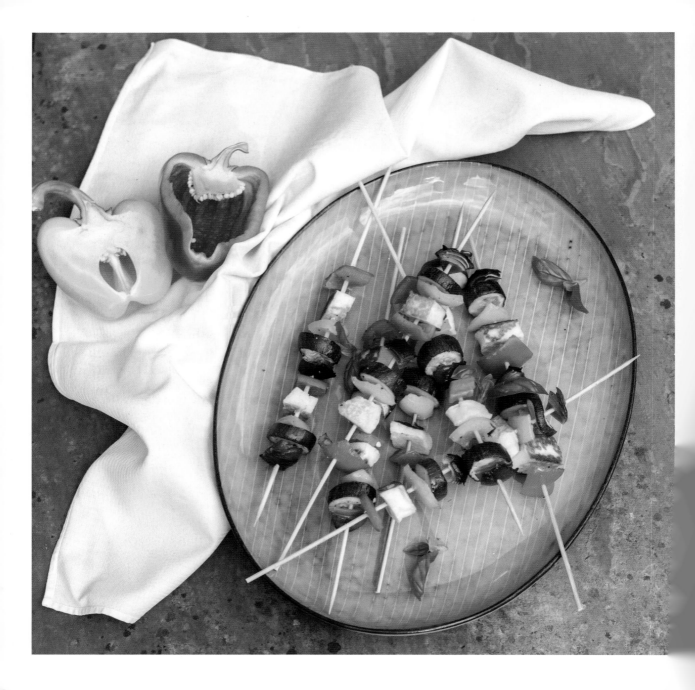

RAINBOW VEGETABLE & HALLOUMI SKEWERS

MAKES 12

- 1 courgette (around 200g)
- 1 red pepper
- 1 yellow pepper
- 1 large red onion (around 150g)
- Olive oil
- Salt and pepper
- 200g halloumi
- sprigs of basil, to serve

You will need

- 12 skewers (if wooden, soak in water for 20 minutes before use to prevent burning)

All these rainbow vegetables on skewers won't do anything to your body's pH I'm afraid, no matter how 'alkaline' they apparently are. That doesn't mean you shouldn't eat them anyway, especially if you're having a barbecue in the sunshine.

Preheat the oven to 200°C fan/220°C conventional/gas mark 7.

Cut the courgette, peppers and onion into chunky cubes and spread them over a baking tray. Drizzle with olive oil, season with salt and pepper, and put them in the oven to roast for around 15 minutes.

Allow the vegetables to cool. In the meantime, cut the halloumi into cubes.

Assemble the skewers: a cube of red pepper, halloumi, yellow pepper, courgette, onion, and repeat once more. Repeat this for each skewer.

Heat a barbecue or griddle pan until very hot, and cook on each side for a few minutes.

Serve immediately with sprig of basil as part of a barbecue feast.

TIP Halloumi goes rubbery quickly when cooled, so only cook these just before you're ready to dish up!

RATATOUILLE QUICHE

SERVES 6-8

- 1 ready rolled shortcrust pastry sheet (320g)
- 1 aubergine (around 200g), sliced into 5mm-thick circles
- 1 green courgette (around 200g), sliced into 5mm-thick circles
- 1 yellow courgette (around 200g), sliced into 5mm-thick circles
- 100ml single cream
- 2 eggs, beaten
- 100g cheddar cheese, grated
- Small bunch of fresh basil, roughly chopped
- Salt and pepper
- 250g tomatoes
- Olive oil

You will need

- A loose-based tart tin approximately 25cm in diameter, greased with olive oil

This is the recipe you need if you're trying to impress. The key is to try to get vegetables with similar diameters, so think long, thin aubergines and wide courgettes. It's a wonderful balance of carbohydrates, fats, protein and includes plenty of vegetables. The cheese is considered 'acidic' so it's a good thing that doesn't matter!

Preheat the oven to 150°C fan/170°C conventional/gas mark 3.

Line the tart tin with pastry and blind bake for 15 minutes. In the meantime, microwave the aubergine and courgettes for 3 minutes.

Make the filling by mixing together the cream, egg, cheese and basil until well combined. Season and pour into the baked pastry case.

Assemble stacks of vegetable: an aubergine slice then tomato then yellow courgette then green. Take each of these and place them at a slight diagonal around the edge of the pastry to form a circle. Then repeat for an inner circle. You should have just enough to cover the whole quiche. Generously season with salt, pepper and olive oil.

Increase the oven temperature to 170°C fan/190°C conventional/gas mark 5.

Place a round piece of baking paper on top and bake for 30 minutes. Then take the paper off and bake for another 20 minutes. Leave to cool for 5 minutes before removing from the tin to serve.

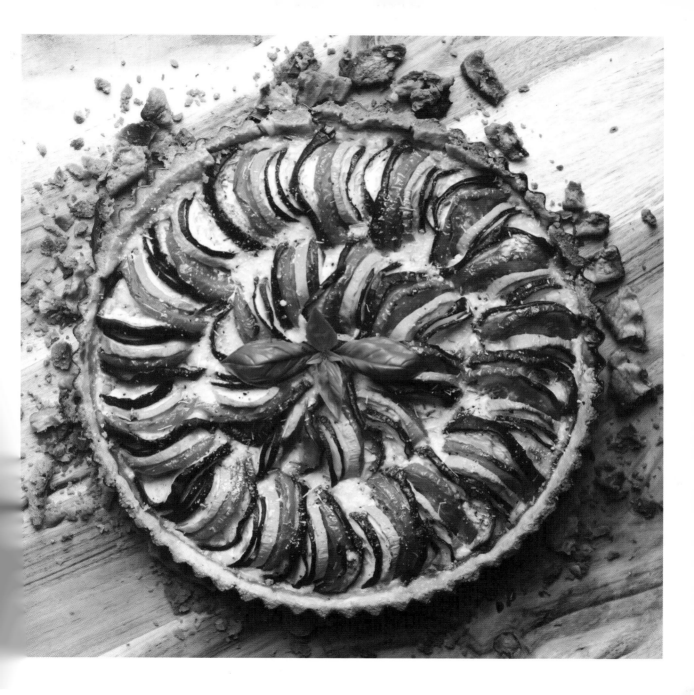

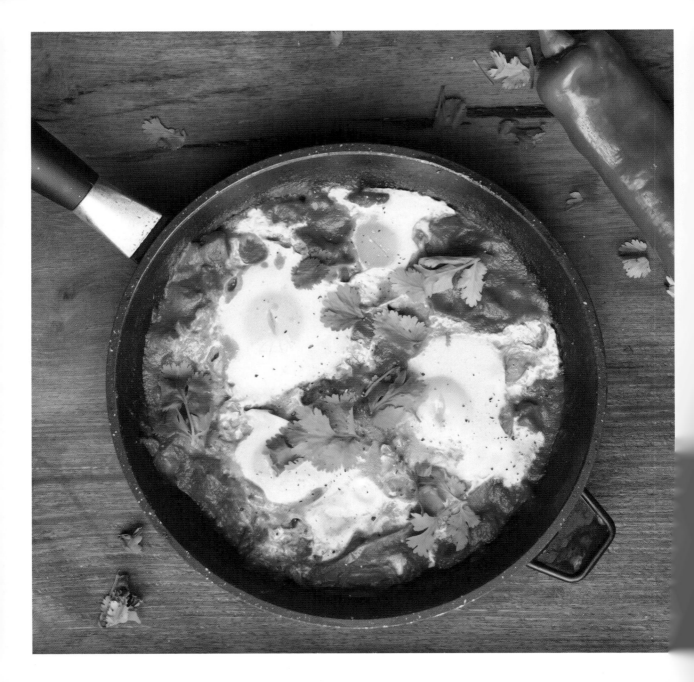

SHAKSHUKA

SERVES 2

- Olive oil
- 1 garlic clove
- 1 red pepper, sliced
- 1 x 400g tin of chopped tomatoes
- Splash of water
- 1 tsp paprika
- ¼ – ½ tsp chilli flakes
- Salt and pepper
- 4 medium eggs
- Fresh coriander, to serve

In true alkaline diet nutribollocks fashion, eggs – a nutritional powerhouse – are on the naughty list. Don't listen to that; eggs are delicious, wonderful things, and are the star of the show in this brunch favourite.

Place a large frying pan over a medium heat and add a splash of olive oil.

Peel and crush the garlic and add it to the pan. Stir for 2 minutes.

Add the sliced peppers and cook for another few minutes. Don't char too much. Add the chopped tomatoes along with a splash of water.

Cook down for 5–10 minutes until a lot thicker. Then season with paprika, chilli flakes, salt and pepper. Taste and adjust the seasoning if necessary.

Make four little wells in the tomato sauce and break an egg into each one. Reduce the heat, and if you have a lid for your pan, place that on. For runny yolks, wait until the egg whites are just cooked, then take off the heat.

Serve with a sprinkling of fresh coriander (unless you hate it) and crusty bread.

Raw foods

THE RAW FOOD MYTH

Of all the different diets and ways of eating out there, some clearly have more evidence to back them up than others. Raw veganism, which deems cooking food to be 'killing' it, is about as restrictive as it gets. On this diet, you can eat nothing but fruits, vegetables, leafy greens, nuts, and seeds. All raw of course.

So does raw veganism have evidence to support it? Nope!

Raw foodism centres around the incorrect belief that uncooked food is intrinsically healthier than cooked food. Although there are inconsistencies within the community about what actually constitutes a raw food diet (what percentage raw does the diet have to be to count? Above what temperature is food no longer 'raw'? [1]), there are some generally agreed upon components:

1. Humans ate raw food and were fine, then we started cooking and everything went horribly wrong.
2. All other animals eat raw food and are healthier than humans, as well as living proportionately longer.
3. Raw food contains 'live' enzymes that are good for you.
4. Cooking food kills it and produces toxins. Cooking food also depletes it of vitamins and phytonutrients.

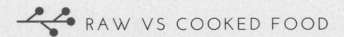 RAW VS COOKED FOOD

Firstly, there is no evidence to suggest humans were healthier when we only ate raw food. Experts believe that cooking likely contributed to human brain expansion, as it reduced the need for large teeth and jaw muscles, thereby allowing larger brain evolution.

Secondly, there's no evidence to suggest that animals are healthier or live proportionately longer than humans. The human lifespan has increased hugely in the last few hundred years thanks to science.

Thirdly, raw food does contain 'live' enzymes, yes. And cooking does denature these enzymes, thereby rendering them non-functional when heated above around 40°C. You know what else denatures enzymes? Your digestive system, duh. Your stomach sits at a comfortable pH of around 2–3 thanks to the production of gastric acids. That's highly acidic, as enzymes such as proteases which break down proteins function optimally in this kind of environment.

Your body can't use plant enzymes; they get broken down in your stomach just like any other protein would, and your body uses the resulting amino acids as building blocks to make other proteins. Your body doesn't 'recruit' plant enzymes for its own use. Essentially, plant enzymes are not going to help you with digestion. Enzymes in some fermented foods such as sauerkraut will actually make it past the stomach intact, but they still contribute negligibly towards our digestion process. Plants use plant enzymes, humans use human enzymes. End of.

Finally, cooking food may 'kill' (if you want to use such dramatic language) the enzymes in food, but that doesn't render the food 'toxic' or a nutritional wasteland. Cooking food can actually remove toxins such as cyanogens or lectins (which you might have come across in the media) and kills bacteria and parasites that could harm you. By cooking food, you're helping avoid food poisoning. In some cases, cooking food can break down some vitamins, yes, but in other cases it makes them more bioavailable (i.e. easier for your body to use). In many cases, cooking breaks down indigestible plant components such as fibres and cell walls, which means better access to the nutrients inside. So, it's not clear-cut and it really depends on the food.

Some water-soluble vitamins, such as B vitamins and vitamin C, leach out from vegetables when boiled. Loss of vitamin C is typically 15–55%, depending on the cooking method [2]. Steaming or boiling generally leads to greater loss of vitamin C compared to microwaving. Polyphenols are often also reduced during cooking. Carrots lose polyphenols when cooked, but the availability of carotenoids (like beta-carotene) increases [3].

Oxalates are compounds found in many plants. They inhibit calcium and iron absorption from foods, so although foods like spinach may be a decent source of both of these, the presence of oxalates in spinach reduces the bioavailability of these nutrients, and your body doesn't use them. However, this mainly applies to raw spinach, as cooking decreases oxalates and therefore increases absorption of iron and calcium [4].

In a similar vein, phytates are commonly found in legumes, grains, nuts and seeds. Phytates provide an energy source for sprouting seeds, as phytase enzymes break down the stored phytates to convert to energy. So they're kind of important to plants. Most phytate is broken down in the stomach and small intestines. But they can bind minerals such as iron or zinc before they are absorbed by the body. Luckily, heating, sprouting and fermenting all reduce the amount of phytates in these foods [5]. Although phytates are often portrayed as 'anti-nutrients', they actually have beneficial effects: consuming foods rich in phytates decreases risk of some cancers and cardiovascular disease [6].

I should probably point out that cooking foods to oblivion or excessively charring foods isn't recommended, but light cooking has some clear health benefits for a lot of foods.

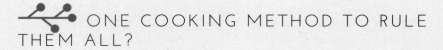

ONE COOKING METHOD TO RULE THEM ALL?

What, then, is the best method for cooking foods? There's boiling, steaming, frying, grilling, baking and microwaving. Ah . . . microwaves. Scaremongers on the internet will argue that microwaves 'nuke' and 'kill' the nutrients in food. Not helpful. Microwave ovens produce microwaves which are waves on the electromagnetic spectrum, along with UV, infrared, X-rays, radio waves and visible light. Microwaves have a higher wavelength than radio waves, but less so than X-rays and even visible light. Microwaves heat food by causing the bonds between water molecules to vibrate, which causes them to warm up. I've seen arguments that this means microwaves can break bonds in our cells. There are three fundamental problems with this argument: firstly, microwave ovens have a casing that prevents waves from escaping. Secondly, microwaves are not powerful enough to break bonds, they can just about make them vibrate. Thirdly, microwaves are all around us all the time anyway, in the form of cosmic microwave background radiation – the energy left over from the big bang. In microwave ovens, these are far more concentrated, which is why they're able to heat up food, but they're contained; they're not going to affect you unless you place yourself inside one while it's on.

Analysis of antioxidants in food after cooking shows that microwaving, baking and grilling produce the smallest losses of nutrients, whereas boiling produces the greatest losses [7], suggesting that the presence of water is the biggest issue. It follows then, that the best cooking method for retaining nutrients is the one that cooks food quickly and uses the least liquid, and microwaving absolutely fits that criteria. But the best cooking method and best way of cooking and eating vegetables is the way that means you'll actually eat them! If you don't have time to bake a potato for an hour in the oven but you have time to microwave it for 10 minutes, then that's the best method. If you find boiled carrots dull but find roasted carrots delicious, then roast them! And if you can easily boil vegetables all together but don't have a steamer, then boil away. What matters in the end is eating the vegetables; if you don't eat them it doesn't matter how healthy they are!

Microwaving, baking and grilling foods result in the least nutrients being lost.

THE MYTHS OF RAW VEGAN DIETS

It's ironic, really, that the rationale for a raw vegan diet tends to be health, as opposed to veganism which is generally adopted for ethical reasons. Many who have adopted it make claims that ailments have been healed and that they have lost incredible amounts of weight by eating a completely or predominantly raw diet. There is very little research on raw veganism, so naturally anecdotes feature prominently.

A raw vegan diet offers no proven health benefits over a vegan or vegetarian diet.

Raw vegan diets are associated with low LDL and triglyceride levels (good), but also lower HDL levels and high homocysteine levels (bad) [8]. There, that's the best I could find to give a balanced 'positive' side. Now let's move on to the downsides.

Vegans in general, raw or not, are at higher risk of B12 deficiency, and B12 supplementation is highly recommended [9]. But tablet supplements aren't seen as 'natural' and 'raw', so supplementation isn't generally encouraged in raw vegan communities. 'Gurus' (ugh) will proudly share their blood test results on YouTube showing their lack of deficiencies, which is great, except you can easily falsify them by simply taking a supplement the day before. Aside from B12, nutritional deficiencies on a raw vegan diet can include vitamin D, selenium, iron, omega-3 and zinc.

Raw vegans may also be at risk of lower bone density mass [10], possibly due to lower calcium and vitamin D intake, as well as the fact that it's associated with being underweight and amenorrhea (loss of periods) [11]. But of course, rather than entertain any possibility of there being downsides to their dietary choice, raw foodists have decided to claim that periods are 'toxins' leaving the body, and that they don't have periods because they are 'pure' and clearly so much better than everyone else. This is bad. Like really bad. And so wrong on so many levels. This is grade A nutribollocks, the finest quality shit to destroy your brain cells. Losing your periods is a sign something is wrong, not that you've reached some special state of 'purity'.

Raw veganism drastically reduces the number of foods you can eat, and variety is key to obtaining all the nutrients we need, as well as feeding a diverse microbiome. A raw vegan diet has no proven health benefits over a vegan or vegetarian diet, but with the added pitfalls of restriction, challenging social situations and potential deficiencies.

Oh, and did I mention that people have died in the care of raw food gurus, both during their retreats and as a result of being told by said gurus to shun conventional medicine in favour of fasting, mono-meals and eating raw? This is not okay. And this is why these kinds of restrictive diets make me angry. I couldn't care less what you choose to eat; it's not my business (unless you pay me to analyse your diet, but even then, I make recommendations and advise, not dictate), but I do have a problem when people make ridiculous claims about curing everything under the sun and venture beyond 'this food is good for you' to 'this diet cures cancer, but only if you give me your money and let me guide you'. Raw foodism is a gateway to a huge host of quack medicine and alternative therapies that don't have a shred of evidence or credibility to their name and can kill people [12].

Right, now that's off my chest, let's talk more about the foods themselves. The following recipes feature a whole host of ingredients that vary in the bioavailability of their nutrients. Some foods are arguably 'healthier' when cooked, some when raw, but that doesn't mean that's the only way you should eat them. The most important thing is to eat your fruits and veggies in a way that means you'll actually enjoy them and be more likely to eat them again, rather than how you 'should' eat them. The following are merely suggestions, not rules.

SOME EXAMPLES

- Tomatoes - contains lycopene which is more bioavailable when cooked
- Butternut squash - contain beta-carotene, lycopene and vitamin C, which all increase when cooked
- Beetroot - doesn't lose its antioxidant activity when cooked
- Spinach - contains calcium and iron which are more bioavailable when cooked
- Citrus fruits - they lose a lot of vitamin C when cooked, so are best eaten raw
- Beans - they contain phytates and lectins which are reduced when cooked and therefore more nutritious
- Potatoes - taste shit when raw but when cooked are a thing of beauty

PIXIE TIP
The best way to eat vegetables is the method you enjoy most – you don't get any benefits by not eating them!

Some foods are more nutritious when cooked, others when raw, but these are not rules to live by, merely suggestions

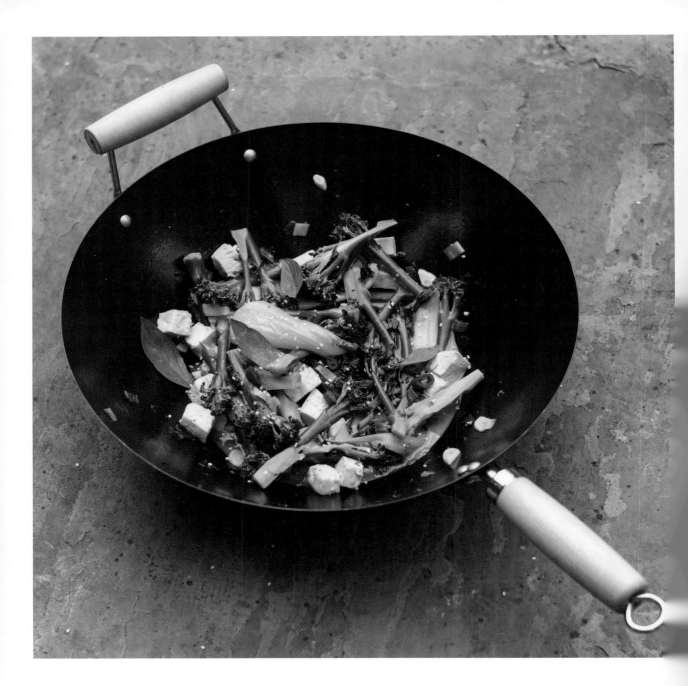

ASIAN STIR-FRIED GREENS WITH TOFU

SERVES 2 AS A MAIN OR 4 AS A SIDE

- 200g tenderstem broccoli (or regular broccoli if you prefer)
- 1 pak choy (around 100g)
- 1 tsp sesame seeds
- Sesame oil
- 2 garlic cloves, peeled and sliced
- 200g smoked tofu, diced
- 2 spring onions, sliced
- ½ fresh red chilli and a few Thai basil leaves (optional)

For the dressing
- 2 tbsp light soy sauce
- 1 tbsp sesame oil (or stir-fry oil)
- 1 tbsp grated ginger
- 1 tbsp lime juice
- 1 tbsp maple syrup, honey or rice syrup

Cooking greens like broccoli in water causes the vitamin C to leach out. By cooking them on very high heat for a short period of time instead, we can preserve more of the nutrients.

Chop the tenderstem broccoli into thirds (or if using regular, chop into bite-sized florets). Separate the pak choy leaves and slice any very big ones.

To make the dressing, mix together the soy sauce, sesame oil, ginger, lime juice and syrup.

Heat a wok over a medium heat and toast the sesame seeds for around 5 minutes. Set aside.

Turn up the heat and add a drizzle of oil.

Add the garlic and tofu and cook for around 5 minutes.

Add the rest of the vegetables along with around half the dressing. Cook for another 5 minutes.

Take off the heat and add the rest of the dressing. Sprinkle the toasted sesame seeds on top along with the chopped chilli and basil leaves (if using).

BEETROOT HUMMUS

SERVES 6-8

- 1 x 400g tin of chickpeas, drained and rinsed
- 250g cooked beetroot
- 1 garlic clove, peeled
- 2 tbsp tahini
- ½ lemon, juiced
- 100ml olive oil
- 2 tsp cumin
- Pinch of salt

Beetroots don't lose antioxidant activity when cooked, which is handy considering they're so much more palatable that way! Plus, it gives dishes like this one the most beautiful pink colour.

Put all the ingredients into a food processor in the order shown.

Blend until smooth.

Taste and adjust the seasoning as necessary.

 TIP This tastes great with my black bean burger on page 227!

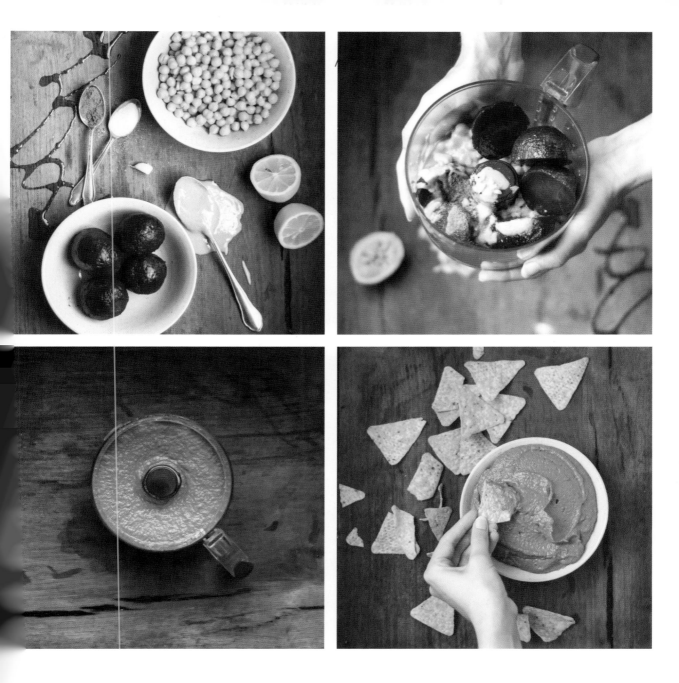

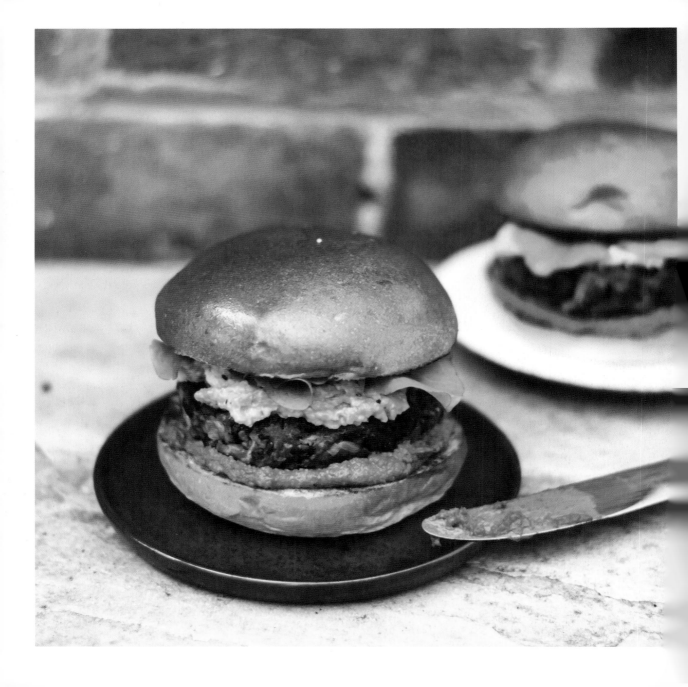

BLACK BEAN BURGER

MAKES 3-4 BURGERS

- 1 x 400g tin of black beans, drained and rinsed
- 1 garlic clove
- 1 onion (around 110g), peeled and very finely diced
- 1 tsp paprika
- 1 tsp cumin
- ¼ tsp chilli powder
- 20g fresh or dried breadcrumbs
- Salt and pepper
- Olive oil
- Burger buns, beetroot hummus (page 224) and mixed slad leaves, to serve

When beans are cooked, both phytates and lectins are reduced, which means more nutrients for you and no toxicity either!

Pat the beans dry and put them into a large bowl. Peel and crush the garlic and add to the bowl along with the diced onion. Add the spices and breadcrumbs and season with salt and pepper.

Mash the mixture together slightly so it starts to coagulate, but leave at least half of the beans whole.

Heat a glug of olive oil in a frying pan over a medium heat.

Form a ball with a third to a quarter of the burger mixture, then gently press until slightly flat. For best results, the burger should be around 2–3cm thick. Bean burgers are more delicate than meat-based burgers, so make sure to form a tight ball of mixture, press it gently and fix any cracks. If the mixture is too crumbly, add an egg or a little oil; if it's too wet, cover your hands with a little flour before shaping the burger.

Fry this burger in the oil over a low heat for a couple of minutes on each side. Flip carefully and only once. Repeat with the remaining burger mix.

Serve in burger buns with beetroot hummus, avocado and mixed salad leaves.

CITRUS, RADISH & WATERCRESS SALAD

SERVES 1 OR 2 AS
A SIDE

- 1 orange (around 160g)
- 1 red or pink grapefruit (around 300g)
- 50g watercress
- 80g radishes, sliced
- ½ sliced avocado, or 30g crumbled feta, or 30g Boursin, or a combination

For the dressing
- 1 tsp wholegrain mustard
- 1 tbsp olive oil
- Pinch of sugar

The vitamin C in citrus fruits would be lost if cooked, so they are best eaten raw to get all the benefits! The cheese or avocado adds a creaminess that complements the sharp citrus nicely. You can add both if you like, I mainly wanted to include a vegan option here!

Segment the orange and grapefruit.

Place the watercress on a plate to create a bed of leaves and arrange the radishes and citrus segments on top.

Add the avocado or sprinkle over the cheese.

Mix together the mustard, olive oil and sugar to create the dressing and drizzle over the salad before serving.

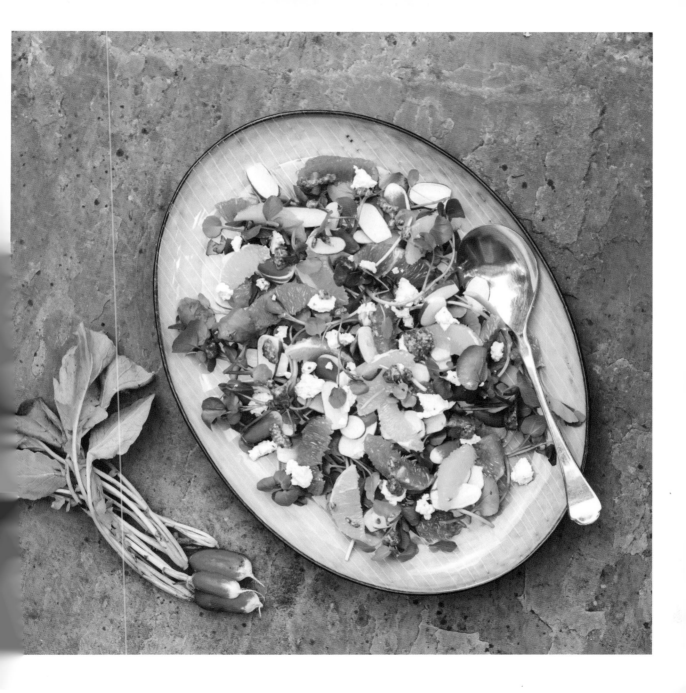

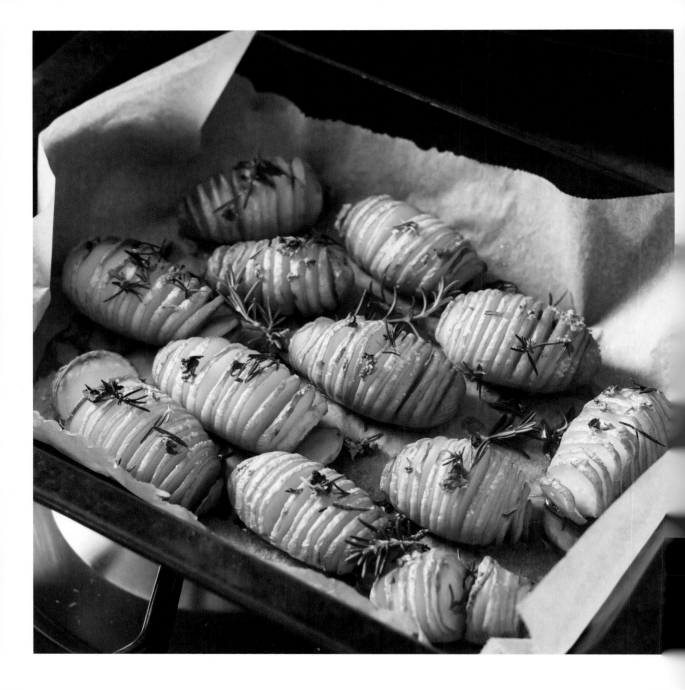

GARLIC & ROSEMARY HASSELBACK POTATOES

SERVES 6-8 AS
A SIDE

- 1kg Charlotte potatoes (these are the best ones for this but feel free to use other types)
- Olive oil
- 2 garlic cloves
- Salt and pepper
- 2 sprigs of fresh rosemary, finely chopped

Potatoes are definitely not meant to be eaten raw. But cooked they become things of beauty! Feel free to scale up or down as much as you like.

Preheat the oven to 220°C fan/240°C conventional/gas mark 9.

Put a potato on to a wooden spoon and cut very thin slices most of the way through the potato. The wooden spoon should stop you from slicing all the way through. Repeat until all the potatoes are finely sliced in this way.

Dip each potato into olive oil briefly and place on a baking tray.

Peel and crush the garlic over the top of the potatoes and sprinkle with salt, pepper and a little of the rosemary.

Roast in the oven for 30–40 minutes, depending on size, then add more fresh rosemary and roast for another 15 minutes.

Serve instead of roast potatoes with a roast dinner, or as a side along with a combination of salads, or any other way you like!

TIP Serve this alongside a Sunday roast instead of standard roast potatoes.

PATATAS BRAVAS WITH ALLIOLI

SERVES 4-6 AS A SIDE

- 600g waxy potatoes, peeled and cut into 2-3cm chunks
- Olive oil
- Salt and pepper
- 1 small onion (around 80g), peeled and finely diced
- 1 x 400g tin of chopped tomatoes
- ½ tsp sugar
- ½ tsp salt
- 1 tsp paprika
- Chilli powder, to taste
- 1 tbsp sherry or wine vinegar (or use lemon juice)

For the allioli
- 1 egg yolk
- 4 garlic cloves
- 1 tbsp lemon juice
- 8 tbsp olive oil
- Salt

Poor potatoes have been demonised by the wellness industry as being 'empty calories', which is far from the truth. Potatoes contain nutrients such as vitamin B6, potassium, copper, vitamin C, manganese, phosphorus, niacin and fibre. But you won't get much out of them unless they're cooked!

Preheat the oven to 200°C fan/220°C conventional/gas mark 7.

Spread the potatoes over a baking tray and drizzle with olive oil. Toss to coat and season. Bake for 45 minutes, until crisp and golden.

To make the tomato sauce, heat a glug of olive oil in a saucepan over a medium heat. Add the onion and cook for around 5-8 minutes.

Add the chopped tomatoes, half a tin of water, sugar, salt, paprika and chilli powder. Stir and leave to gently simmer for around 20 minutes. When done, remove from the heat and stir in the vinegar.

To make the allioli, place the egg yolk, garlic and lemon juice in a food processor. Whizz until blended, then slowly drizzle in the olive oil over the course of a couple of minutes until it becomes thick and creamy. Season with salt.

I prefer to serve the potatoes and the sauces separately, or you can spoon the tomato sauce on top and serve the allioli on the side for those who can't handle the heat (like me)!

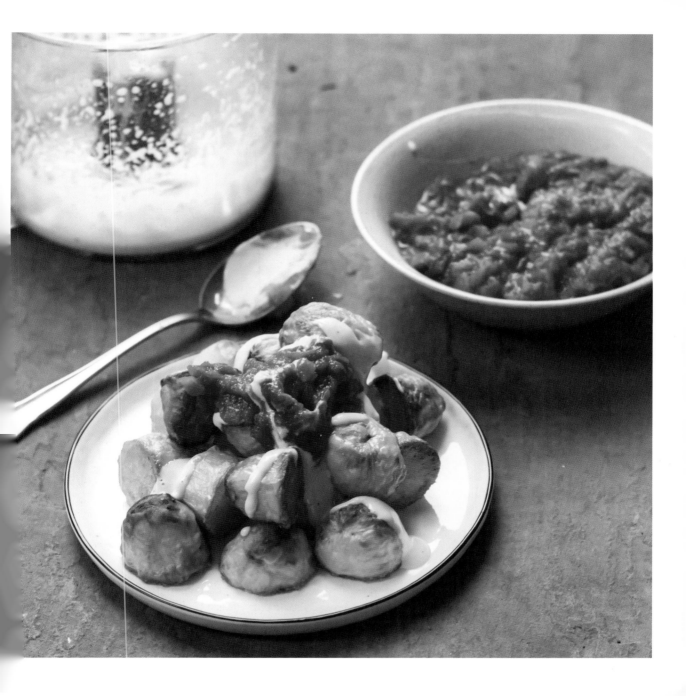

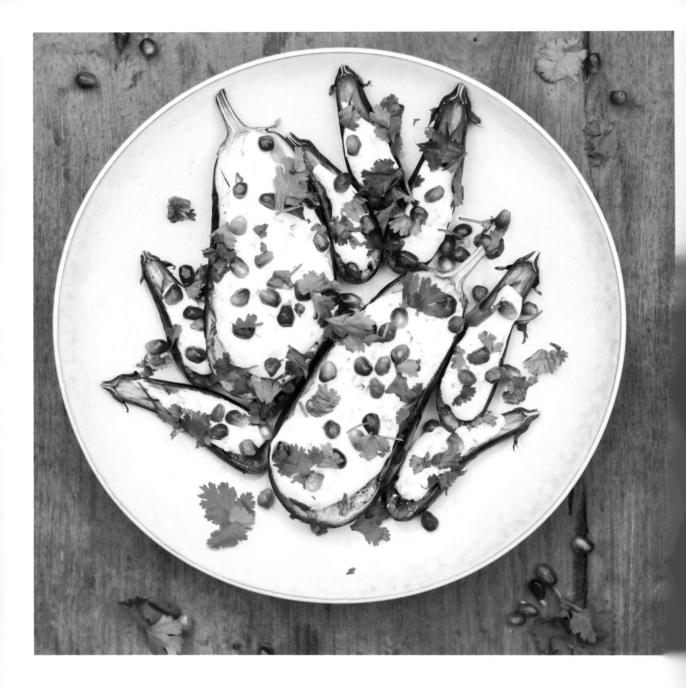

ROASTED AUBERGINE WITH YOGHURT & POMEGRANATE

SERVES 4

- 2 large aubergines (around 600g)
- Olive oil
- Salt and pepper
- 200g Greek yoghurt
- ½ lemon, juiced
- 2 tbsp finely chopped chives
- 50g pomegranate seeds
- Fresh coriander leaves, to serve

Raw aubergine contains the toxin solamine which can cause gut problems. But don't panic, you'd have to eat over thirty of them in one go for it to be a problem. Still, best to eat them cooked anyway, and luckily they taste better that way too.

Preheat the oven to 200°C fan/220°C conventional/gas mark 7.

Cut the aubergines in half lengthways and score the flesh in a criss-cross pattern. Place on a lined baking tray, drizzle with olive oil and season with salt and pepper.

Roast in the oven for around 15–20 minutes, until soft all the way through.

In the meantime, mix together the yoghurt, lemon juice, finely chopped chives and a pinch of salt and pepper.

When the aubergine halves are ready, spoon the yoghurt mixture on top and sprinkle with pomegranate seeds and fresh coriander.

TIP Why not serve with either the greens and beans salad on page 170 or the roasted tomato salad on page 236?

ROASTED TOMATO SALAD

SERVES 4 AS A SIDE

- Olive oil
- 400g small tomatoes (ideally a range of colours and sizes)
- 40g rocket
- 10g pine nuts
- Balsamic vinegar
- Salt and pepper

Tomatoes are most often eaten raw, but when cooked the lycopene is much more bioavailable, which means you get more nutrients from them!

Heat a griddle pan over a medium heat and drizzle with olive oil.

Halve the tomatoes lengthways. Place on the griddle pan flesh-side down, until gently seared.

Meanwhile, wash and dry the rocket and arrange on a serving plate. Place the cooked tomatoes on top, seared side up.

Sprinkle the pine nuts over the top.

Drizzle with balsamic vinegar and season with salt and pepper.

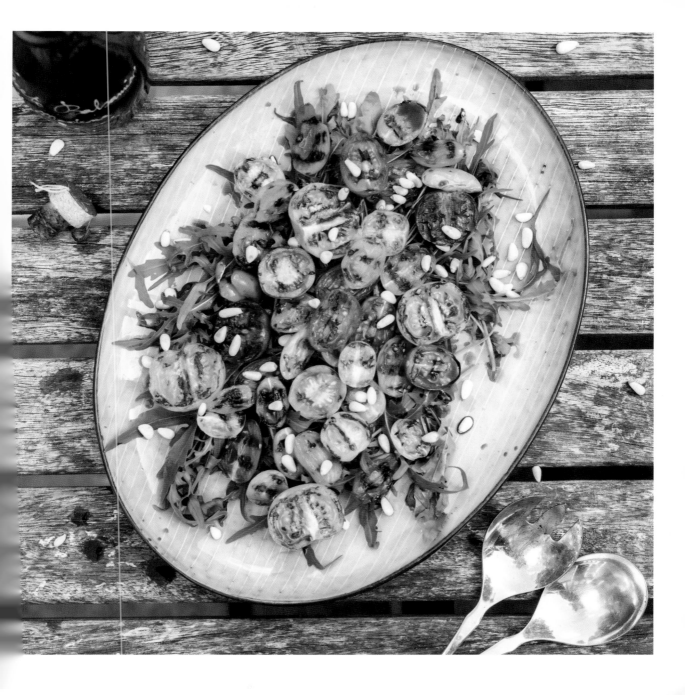

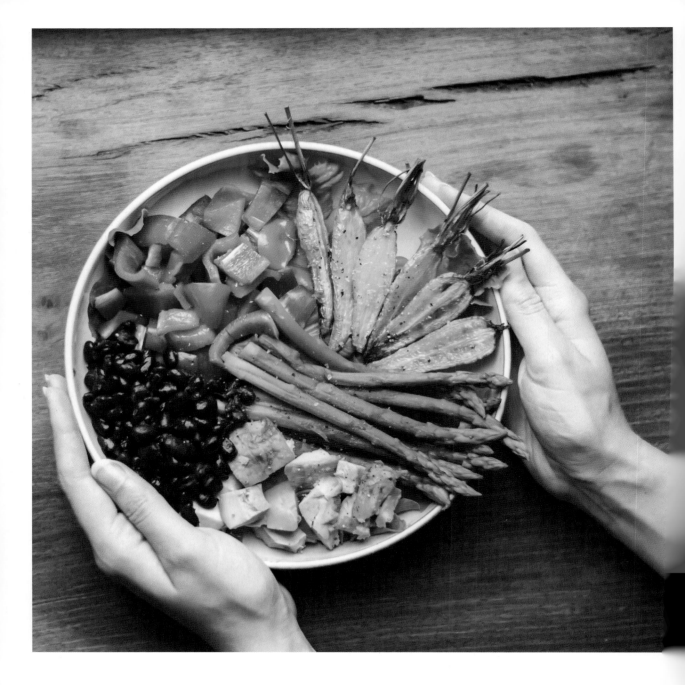

SPRING/SUMMER PIXIE PLATE

SERVES 1

- 80g carrots
- Olive oil
- Salt and pepper
- 80g asparagus
- Handful of salad leaves, such as spinach or rocket
- 60g red pepper, roughly chopped
- ½ avocado, cubed
- 80g cooked black beans

My Pixie Plates have become my signature style on Instagram. They contain a mix of raw and cooked vegetables, according to your liking. They're a great way to get a rainbow of delicious foods into your body!

Preheat the oven to 200°C fan/220°C conventional/gas mark 7.

Cut the carrots in halves or quarters, depending on size. Place on a baking tray, drizzle with olive oil and season with salt and pepper. Roast in the oven for 20 minutes.

Snap off the woody ends of the asparagus and boil in salted water for 5 minutes, steam for 5 minutes, or microwave on high for 3 minutes.

Assemble everything on a plate: salad leaves first, then arrange the rest of the ingredients on top. Season everything with salt and pepper and drizzle with a dressing of your choice.

AUTUMN/WINTER PIXIE PLATE

SERVES 1

- 100g butternut squash, peeled and diced
- 80g aubergine, sliced
- Olive oil
- Salt and pepper
- 40g puy lentils (80g cooked)
- 80g tenderstem broccoli
- 100g tomatoes
- Handful of salad leaves such as spinach or rocket

This plate is another perfect example of how using a mix of raw and cooked ingredients makes for a perfectly delicious balanced meal! Take the butternut squash, for example: the beta-carotene, lycopene and vitamin C in squash are all increased when roasted!

Preheat the oven to 200°C/220°C conventional/gas mark 6.

Spread the butternut squash and aubergine over a baking tray in a single layer, drizzle with olive oil and season with salt and pepper. Roast in the oven for 20 minutes, until soft.

If using raw lentils, cook these in boiling salted water (or with ¼ vegetable stock cube) for 20 minutes.

Cut the broccoli pieces in half. Boil in salted water for 4 minutes, steam for 5 minutes, or microwave on high for 2–3 minutes.

If using cherry tomatoes, cut each one in half. If using larger tomatoes, dice.

Assemble everything on a plate: salad leaves first, then arrange the rest of the ingredients on top.

Season the tomatoes with salt and pepper and add a dressing of your choice.

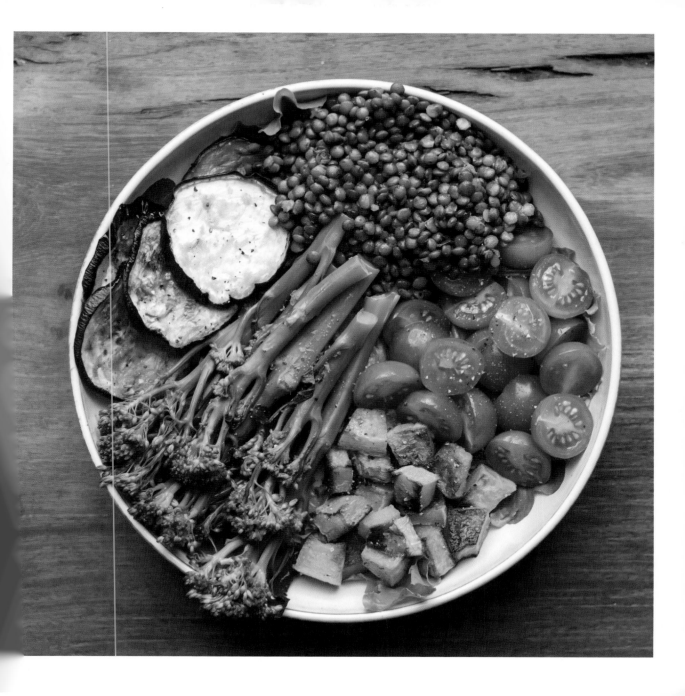

sugar

THE REFINED SUGAR MYTH

I hope you're ready for a bit of biochemistry with this one. Nothing too intense, don't worry, but to try to understand the nature of sugar and why I can't believe this myth is still in existence, we have to go right down to the chemical structures.

We have an epidemic of misunderstanding around sugar, which in itself doesn't sound terrible; I mean we all know that eating too much sugar isn't good for us, and we've been told over and over how it's hiding in everything we eat. But when you see phrases such as 'sugar is poison' and 'sugar is addictive' or see people genuinely terrified of eating a banana or of putting a teaspoon of white table sugar in their coffee, then we have a problem.

I've seen bloggers argue that sugar from natural sources, such as coconut sugar, is superior to white table sugar, conveniently forgetting that white table sugar comes from sugar cane or beets. Definitely both plants. Definitely both natural. 'Oh, but it's so processed that you can barely call it natural anymore'. Firstly, that's irrelevant because it still comes from natural sources, and secondly, the same argument can be applied to the 'natural flavourings' you see in so many health products, but people don't seem to have a problem with those.

SUGAR BIOCHEMISTRY

Sugars are simple carbohydrates (go back to Chapter 2 to refresh your memory if you need to); simple because they are small structures that are more quickly and easily absorbed than complex carbohydrates. The main ones we're interested in are monosaccharides and disaccharides. Monosaccharides are solo sugars (mono = one), such as glucose and fructose. Disaccharides are two monosaccharides joined together (di = two), such as sucrose.

Sucrose

CH_2OH H O H OH H OH H OH CH_2OH O H H HO CH_2OH OH H

When sucrose enters the body, an enzyme breaks it down into glucose and fructose. If you remember from Chapter 2, glucose and fructose are metabolised differently in the body due to their different structures.

Glucose, fructose and sucrose are all sugars. Lactose is a sugar too, but that's a different story. For some unknown reason, many bloggers decide to categorise sugars differently to the government guidelines. Rather than sorting them into intrinsic and free (i.e. added) sugars, they decide to sort them into refined and unrefined sugars. This, as I'm about to demonstrate, makes very little sense.

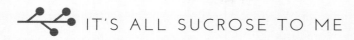

IT'S ALL SUCROSE TO ME

So why the biochemistry lesson? Well, sucrose is what makes table sugar sweet. In fact, table sugar (white, brown, caster, etc.) is essentially 100% pure sucrose. But how does this compare to 'unrefined' sugars, such as coconut sugar and maple syrup?

TABLE SUGAR/WHITE SUGAR/CASTER SUGAR	
Made from	Sugarcane or sugar beets. Involves extraction with hot water, concentration of the syrups, crystallisation of solid sugar and purification.
Composition	Sucrose (100%)
Micronutrients	None

COCONUT SUGAR	
Made from	The sap of the coconut plant. Involves extraction and heating to remove water.
Composition	Sucrose (around 85%), glucose (3-5%), fructose (3-5%), moisture and fibre (3-4%), protein (1%)
Micronutrients	May contain zinc, iron, calcium and potassium

MAPLE SYRUP	
Made from	The sap of maple trees, heated to concentrate it into syrup
Composition	Varies. Carbohydrate (67%, mainly sucrose, some fructose and glucose) and water (32-33%)
Micronutrients	Approximately 1%. Mainly vitamin B2 and manganese, plus a variety of flavour compounds

HIGH FRUCTOSE CORN SYRUP (HFCS)	
Made from	Derived from corn, intended as a substitute for table sugar that is more easily transported and more stable.
Composition	Carbohydrate (76%, of which 55% is fructose and 45% is glucose) and water (24%)
Micronutrients	None

AGAVE NECTAR	
Made from	The juice from the agave plant, filtered, heated and concentrated.
Composition	Varies. Fructose (approximately 55-65%), glucose (approximately 12%), water (approximately 23%)
Micronutrients	Varies. A darker colour means more plant minerals

Overall, the main difference between 'refined' and 'unrefined' sugars is small.

RICE SYRUP	
Made from	Culturing cooked rice to break down starch into sugars and concentrating it.
Composition	Glucose and glucose chains (approximately 85%), water (approximately 15%)
Micronutrients	Some, but also arsenic

Overall, the main differences between table sugar, coconut sugar, maple syrup and HFCS are small. They all have similar amounts of glucose and fructose in them (remembering that sucrose is 50% glucose and 50% fructose). The main difference between them is the amount of micronutrients, and in cases like coconut sugar, a little fibre. However, the level of micronutrients in all of these is around 1% maximum, which means you'd have to eat huge amounts to get meaningful amounts of nutrients from them. And even if you did eat enough to get significant nutrients, the beneficial effects would be cancelled out by the large amount of sugar you've consumed. For example, 100g of maple syrup has 10% of your daily calcium requirements. But you'd also be eating 20 teaspoons of added sugar (assuming 1 tsp = 5g), which is four times your recommended daily maximum. Compare that with 100g cow's milk, which offers you 18% of your calcium needs and no added sugar, or 100g kale, which offers you 15% of your daily calcium needs and definitely no added sugar. I know, I'm defending kale, who'd have thought?! Overall, the differences between table sugar and the sugars wellness bloggers recommend are so small that direct substitution in a healthy balanced diet wouldn't lead to any health benefits.

Agave and rice syrup are a bit more different, to be fair – agave is high in fructose and low in glucose, whereas rice syrup is pure glucose – but that doesn't mean you should be scared of or go nuts on either of them. The point I really want to emphasise here is that wellness bloggers claim that 'unrefined' sugars are healthier and more nutritious. This simply is not the case.

ARTIFICIAL SWEETENERS

Artificial sugars, or 'zero calorie' sweeteners, are an entirely different story. They have a completely different biochemical composition to sucrose. Let's focus on three of the main artificial sweeteners in use in the UK: stevia, sucralose and aspartame.

Stevia is extracted from the leaves of the Stevia plant and is highly purified. Its sweetness comes from steviol glycosides, which are up to 150 times sweeter than sucrose, and have a much more complicated chemical structure.

Steviol glycoside

Sucralose is derived from sucrose and as such looks similar, but is mostly left undigested by the body (hence 'zero calorie'). It's around 600 times sweeter than sucrose.

Sucalrose

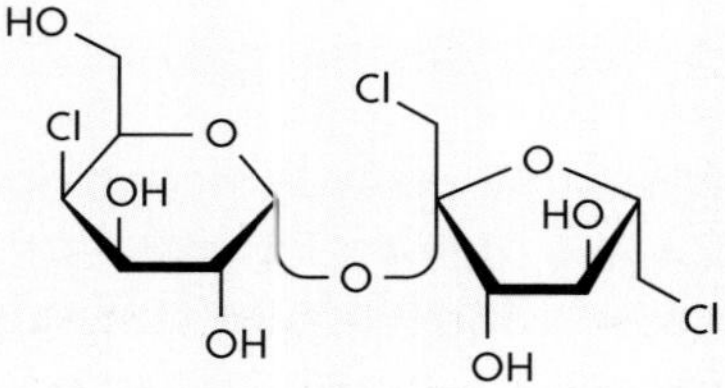

Aspartame is actually two amino acids joined together that trick your taste buds into sensing sweetness. It looks nothing like sucrose and is around 200 times sweeter.

Aspartame

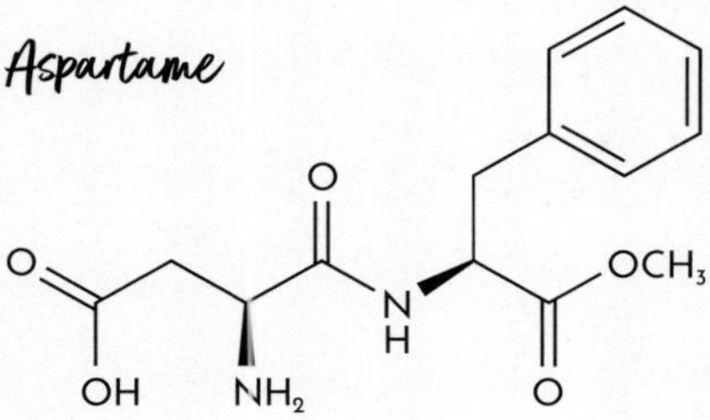

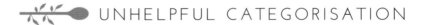 ## UNHELPFUL CATEGORISATION

Categorising sugars into 'processed' and 'unprocessed' is not only unhelpful, it's misleading and potentially damaging. Demonising table sugar and hailing maple syrup as being 'healthy' or 'good for you', doesn't make sense. Besides, if you haven't already noticed, they're all processed in some way. Maple syrup doesn't come out of the tree looking like that; it comes out as a sap that has to be filtered and concentrated (though the sap is now available to buy as 'maple water'). Similarly, you won't find coconut sugar spilling out when you cut open a coconut palm. That's not how it works. They are all processed, some just slightly more than others, so dichotomising them into two groups of 'refined' and 'unrefined' or 'processed' and 'unprocessed' is missing the point entirely.

Describing sugars as either processed or natural makes no sense either. All of the above fall into both categories. Whether it's sugarcane, corn, coconut palms, maple trees, rice or agave plants, they all come from natural sources: plants. It's a ridiculously unhelpful classification; in fact, it's so pointless it doesn't even dichotomise. All these sugars are processed and all these sugars are natural.

The government guidelines, outlined in the SACN (Scientific Advisory Committee on Nutrition) report on carbohydrates in 2015, group all of the above sugars into one category: free sugars. They say, 'Free sugars are those added to food or those naturally present in honey, syrups and unsweetened fruit juices, but exclude lactose in milk and milk products' [1]. It also excludes sugars found in intact fruits and vegetables. It's recommended that we limit free sugar intake to no more than 5% of total daily calories, regardless of whether it's from table sugar or maple syrup. That's the equivalent of 5 teaspoons of table sugar or 5 teaspoons of maple syrup or 5 teaspoons of coconut sugar. Same shit, different name.

GLYCAEMIC NUTRIBOLLOCKS

Surely, if maple syrup was so much better for you, it wouldn't be put into the same category as table sugar? Oh, but what about glycaemic index (GI)? Bloggers love to claim that coconut sugar has a lower GI value than table sugar, which makes it healthier. The glycaemic index of a food is a measure of the effect it has on blood sugar levels. Generally, more glucose means a higher GI value, and more fibre means a lower GI value, because it slows release. Coconut sugar has slightly more fibre than table sugar, so it is considered to be lower GI, but that's not the complete picture. What may matter more than glycaemic index is actually glycaemic load (GL), as GL takes into account the amount of carbohydrate in a food, and as such is a more reliable predictor of the effects of food on blood sugar levels. A good example is watermelon, which has a high GI value due to the fruit sugars present. But each serving of watermelon is 92% water, leaving very little carbohydrate per serving, so it has a low GL. Similarly, because fructose is a carbohydrate that has a low GI value, sweeteners like agave which are very high in fructose have a low GI value but a higher GL. It also means that coconut sugar has the same GL as white table sugar.

Another common myth is that eating sugar triggers an insulin spike, causing your body to store fat. The first part of this is absolutely true; when your blood sugar levels go up it causes insulin to be released. High insulin levels in the blood is the signal for your cells to take up glucose from the blood into cells. That's definitely not the same as 'storing fat', as this glucose can be used for anything from energy production to glycogen storage. Glycogen, not fat. Glucose is the body's preferred energy source, so it will only store this as fat if there's too much floating around and you don't have use for it. And even then, I don't just mean using it to fuel exercise, I mean using it to fuel all basic biological functions that keep you alive. Every move you make requires energy.

The evidence shows that high levels of sugar consumption is associated with greater risk of tooth decay and development of type 2 diabetes. But eating a little bit of sugar isn't going to kill you; in fact it'll probably make you miserable if you don't have any – sweet treats make you happy and are associated with special occasions.

In wellness, white sugar is seen as the 'devil'. Once upon a time, its purity made it highly sought after, now its purity makes it too 'clinical', too far removed from nature. The myth that white sugar is bleached remains to this day, despite the fact that this wouldn't pass food safety regulations. In the UK, white sugar generally comes from sugar beets, whereas brown sugar generally comes from sugar cane, and it retains some of the molasses which gives it its brown colour. White sugar isn't 'bleached' brown sugar; that's just how it looks when it's purified from sugar beet.

Scaring people out of eating sugar might be beneficial for some, but to others it can be incredibly psychologically damaging. But scaring them out of eating table sugar in favour of maple syrup is just another way the wellness industry is taking your money for no good reason. Maple syrup, agave, rice syrup and coconut sugar are all considerably more expensive than table sugar and this feeds that sense of elitism and exclusivity that comes with wellness.

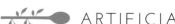 ## ARTIFICIAL SWEETENERS

Artificial sweeteners often get a bad rep simply for being artificial. People assume that because they're artificial they must be bad. I'm just going to go ahead and assume that by now it's sunk in that this argument is irrelevant and focus on more important arguments for and against.

All three of these artificial sweeteners have been approved for use in the

EU, which means they've undergone a very rigorous safety assessment by the European Food Safety Authority (EFSA). Stevia was approved for use in 2012 after a comprehensive analysis that concluded it to be safe [2]. A review of evidence in 2000 found that sucralose is safe for human consumption, is not harmful to the immune system, doesn't cause cancer and doesn't significantly affect blood sugar levels [3]. Aspartame has been the subject of much controversy, but was concluded to be safe after a comprehensive review of the evidence in 2013 [4]. In addition, a study of almost half a million people found that aspartame doesn't increase the risk of leukaemia, lymphoma or brain cancer [5]. I'd trust that over rat studies any day.

Arguments for the use of artificial sweeteners:
- Deemed safe for human consumption
- Doesn't increase the risk of tooth decay
- May not increase the risk of type 2 diabetes (still uncertain)

Arguments against the use of artificial sweeteners:
- Sometimes has a bitter aftertaste
- No major effect on bodyweight (if that's your goal) [6]
- May have negative effects on the gut microbiome (but not clear yet as studies are in mice, needs more research) [7]

The research into the link between artificial sweeteners, appetite stimulation and weight gain is currently inconsistent [8], and more research in this area is definitely needed. But what is clear is that the current research suggests that these sweeteners are safe to consume. It was initially thought they would help people consume less added sugar, thereby reducing overall calorie intake leading to weight loss. However, that doesn't seem to be the case, and emerging evidence suggests that because these sweeteners provide a sweet taste without actually providing energy (in calories), it may increase cravings for sweet foods that do provide energy – i.e. sucrose. This is shown by the fact there's actually no significant difference in energy intake between those who consume sugar-sweetened beverages and artificially sweetened beverages [9], which means they're also just as at risk of type 2 diabetes.

Overall, the argument of whether sweeteners are 'bad for you' seems to be context-dependent and not black and white. If you like your morning coffee sweet, then choosing a sweetener over sucrose might be a good option. But if the alternative to sweetener is nothing sweet at all, then great, you're a stronger human being than I am (I have a very sweet tooth). Baking is a different situation again, as texture and consistency matter as much as flavour, and you just can't replace the beauty of creaming butter and sugar together. Plus, some sweeteners are unstable at high temperatures and so may react with other ingredients.

MORE ADDICTIVE THAN COCAINE?

Is sugar addictive? Medically, a substance is addictive if it (1) causes long-term chemical changes in the brain, (2) causes severe compulsion to consume it, (3) leads to tolerance and (4) causes dependence leading to withdrawal symptoms.

Sugar does activate the reward system and lights up pleasure centres in the brain, causing dopamine release just like drugs. However, cuddling kittens or puppies also activates the reward system, but no one is arguing that's addictive. From an evolutionary perspective, it makes complete sense that we have an inherent desire to eat food; it's essential for survival. Cravings are also different from addiction. We might crave sugar because it's a quick, convenient energy source and because our brains run on glucose. That doesn't mean we're addicted to it. Sugar crashes and cravings are also not the same as withdrawal symptoms, because sugar crashes are due to blood sugar levels dropping, and can be 'cured' by eating pretty much any food; it doesn't have to be sugar. This is quite different from a chemical dependency on drugs, where only the drug can satisfy the craving and cure the withdrawal symptoms. You can't tackle heroin withdrawal symptoms by giving someone ibuprofen. You can't tackle alcohol addiction with soft drinks. But you can raise your blood sugar levels by eating a steak, which contains no sugar at all.

Currently, food addiction is reliant on rat studies, subjective reports and anecdotal evidence. A lot of rat studies rely on depriving them of food for twelve hours, then giving them large amounts of sugar solution. They 'binge' on it because they learn to expect periods of hunger [10]. There was also a study where rats preferred sugar to cocaine [11], leading to a flurry of news headlines that 'sugar is more addictive than cocaine!'. Scary stuff. But this is in rats. How applicable is this to humans?

A review of the evidence in humans and rats found little evidence to support the idea of sugar addiction in humans. And even in rats, the 'addictive' behaviours are argued to only occur due to the restrictive and intermittent access to sugar – basically encouraging restricting and bingeing behaviour – rather than a chemical addiction [12]. These studies have been conducted under conditions that don't resemble typical human environments, as we're generally exposed to sugar and food all the time, so it's hard to argue that they would be applicable to us. Rats preferring sugar to cocaine could also simply be them choosing the lesser of two evils – maybe rats experience a comedown after cocaine too? Overall, it seems that not only are we as humans not addicted to sugar, but the rats aren't either.

Leading experts conclude that 'sugar addiction' doesn't have the evidence to support it. And think about it, when was the last time you saw someone

There is little evidence to support the idea of sugar addiction in humans.

spooning pure sugar into their mouth? You don't see it! What you see instead is that people are more likely to overeat on foods that are high in sugar, fat and starch, such as a donut or cake. These foods are appealing to us from an evolutionary perspective as they tend to be highly palatable and energy-dense.

Researchers also argue that calling it 'food addiction' isn't a good idea, and I would agree, because it encourages people to think their diet is out of their control, it attaches stigma in a society that already has a serious issue with weight bias, and it promotes unhealthy avoidance behaviours (going 'cold turkey') around food. Unlike drugs or alcohol, our brains need carbohydrates like glucose in order to function; it's not optional. You need food to survive, and 99.9% of the time that involves some glucose, some fructose (from fruit) and even some sucrose. You can't be addicted to something that you need to live. So next time you see someone spouting sugar addiction bullshit, give them a dose of science smackdown.

THE SWEET, SWEET TRUTH

The take-home message is this: if you want to use artificial sweeteners as a replacement for sugar in your coffee then go for it, and if you don't, then that's okay too. Just please don't argue that it's simply because 'sugar is natural so it's better'. Remember, individual studies can only tell us so much, and it's the collective overall picture that matters, so don't be put off by scaremongering rat and mice studies. Unless you're a mouse of course.

If you're baking with sugar, then choose the type based on consistency and flavour, not nutrition, as they all count as free sugars and the nutritional differences are insignificant. That's exactly what I'm going to do in this next set of recipes. You'll find everything from golden syrup and maple syrup to caster sugar and even stevia. Because when it comes to sugar, context matters most.

Categorising sugars into "refined" and "unrefined" is not only unhelpful, it's misleading and potentially damaging. All these sugars are processed, and all these sugars are natural

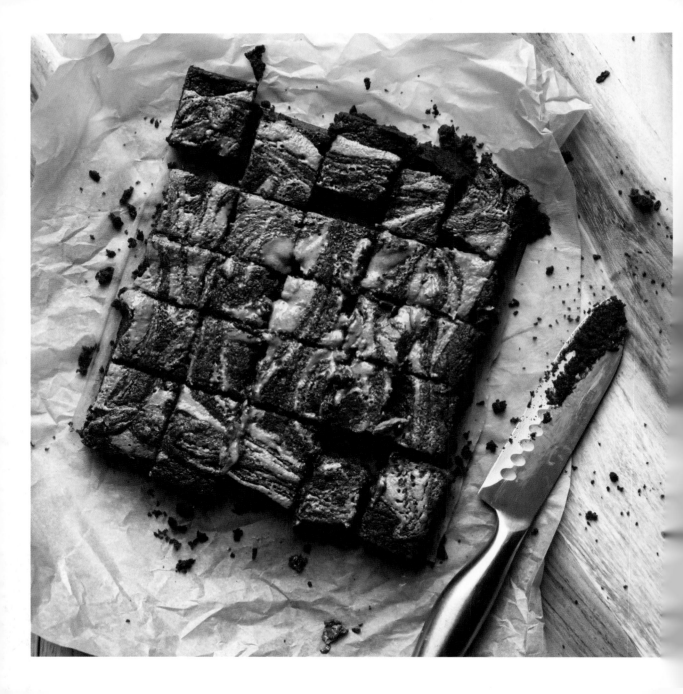

ALMOND BUTTER SWIRLED BROWNIES

MAKES 25 SMALL OR 16 LARGER BROWNIES

- 200g unsalted butter
- 200g dark chocolate
- 250g caster sugar
- 3 medium eggs, beaten
- ½ tsp vanilla bean paste
- Pinch of salt
- 100g plain flour
- 100g salted almond butter (or use unsalted almond butter and add salt)

You will need
- A 20x20cm brownie tin

The best brownies aren't made with sweet potato, cauliflower, aubergine or whatever fresh hell people come up with next. If you have a brownie craving, those things just won't satisfy you. What you really need are these. They have chocolate, sugar, gluten . . . the works.

Preheat the oven to 160°C /180°C conventional/ gas mark 3.

Melt the butter and chocolate together in the microwave or in a heatproof bowl over a saucepan of gently simmering water.

Stir in the sugar, eggs, vanilla bean paste and salt. Stir in the flour.

Line the brownie tin with baking paper and pour in the mixture.

Dollop over the almond butter and swirl the mixture together.

Bake in the oven for around 35 minutes, until just baked and super gooey.

Leave to cool for 15 minutes before cutting into squares.

TIP Not a fan of almond butter? Substitute your favourite nut butter or just leave it out entirely. Only have a loaf tin? Simply halve the mixture or bake in two batches.

BANANA BREAD

SERVES 8-12

- 300g plain flour
- 1 tsp baking powder
- 1 tsp bicarbonate of soda
- 1 tsp ground cinnamon
- Pinch of salt
- 2 eggs, beaten (use 6 tbsp aquafaba (chickpea water) to make it vegan)
- 100g maple syrup
- 6 tbsp olive oil
- 1 tsp vanilla bean paste or vanilla extract
- 50ml milk (oat milk works well too)
- 3 large, very ripe bananas (around 250-300g)
- Optional extras: 150g frozen berries or 150g chocolate chips
-

You will need

- A 1.5 litre loaf tin

For super moist banana bread, the combination of liquid sweeteners and spotty, ripe bananas is key. The extra flavour maple syrup gives over other sweeteners like rice syrup makes it my syrup of choice here. This is probably the sweet recipe with the lowest added sugar in the book! My favourite way to make this is with frozen blueberries, but other berries or chocolate chips work well too.

Preheat the oven to 180°C fan/200°C conventional/gas mark 6.

Mix together the dry ingredients in a bowl (flour, baking powder, bicarbonate of soda, cinnamon and salt).

Mix together the wet ingredients in a separate bowl (eggs, maple syrup, olive oil, vanilla bean paste or extract and milk).

Mash the bananas and add to the wet ingredients. Add the wet mixture to the dry.

Add the frozen berries or chocolate chips, if using.

Pour into a 1.5 litre loaf tin lined with baking paper or greased with a little oil. Bake in the oven for around 45 minutes, until an inserted toothpick comes out clean.

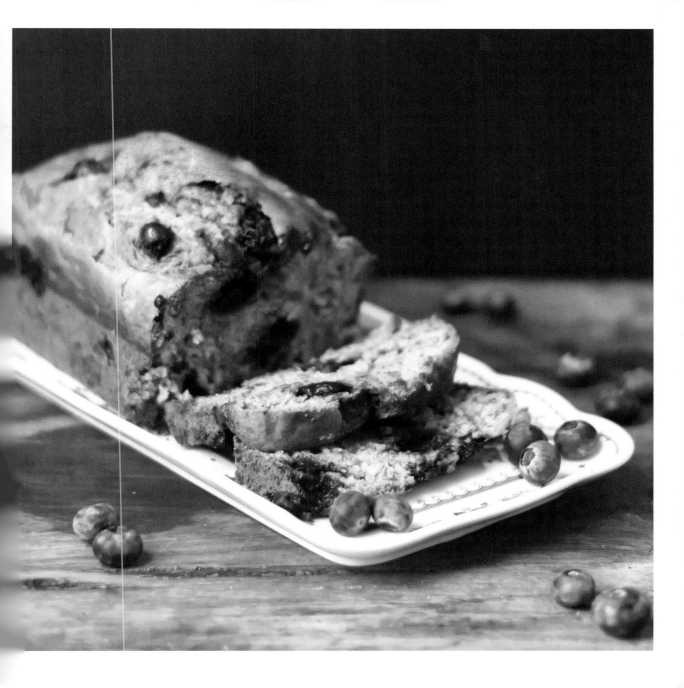

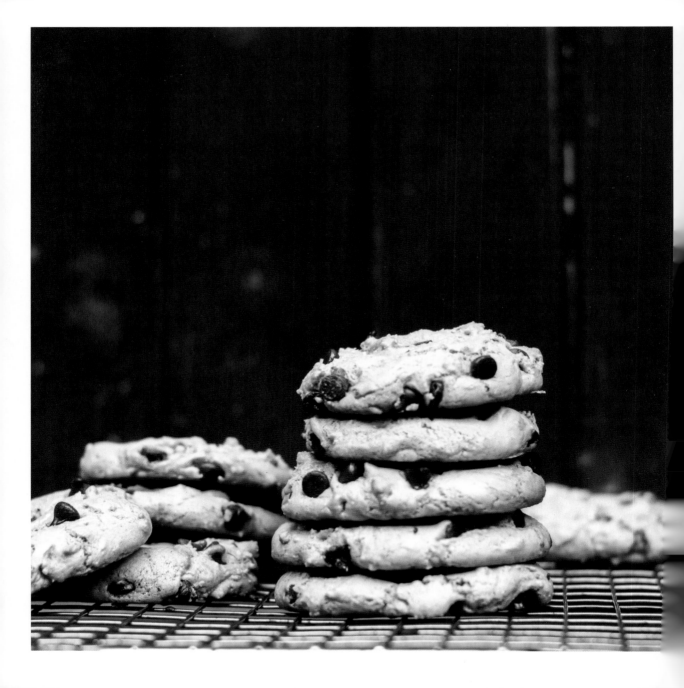

CHOCOLATE CHIP COOKIES

MAKES 10-12 LARGE COOKIES OR 15 SMALLER ONES

- 6 tbsp olive oil
- 150g brown sugar
- 1 medium egg, beaten (use 4 tbsp aquafaba (chickpea water) to make it vegan)
- 1 tsp vanilla bean paste
- ½ tsp bicarbonate of soda
- Pinch of salt
- 200g plain flour
- 100g dark chocolate chips

I like my cookies slightly crunchy on the outside but soft and chewy on the inside. That's why this recipe uses brown sugar, as it helps provide the deliciously chewy texture that makes cookies so enticing!

Preheat the oven to 180°C fan/200°C conventional/gas mark 6.

Mix the oil, sugar, egg and vanilla bean paste together in a bowl.

Add the bicarbonate of soda and salt.

Slowly mix in the flour, a little at a time.

Stir in the chocolate chips.

Form 10-12 tablespoon-sized mounds or 15 smaller ones on a lined baking tray.

Bake in the oven for 12-15 minutes, until barely cooked and still soft to touch. If you've made 15 smaller cookies, bake for 12 minutes max, and if you've made 10-12 larger ones, test them at 12 minutes and bake for 15 minutes max.

Leave to cool for another 15 minutes before touching or moving them.

TIP I actually prefer the texture of the vegan version of these, so give them a try!

CINNAMON ROLLS

MAKES 12 ROLLS

- 240ml warm milk (any kind)
- 1 x 7g sachet of dried yeast
- 2 tbsp granulated sugar
- 1 tsp salt
- 45g butter, softened
- 1 large egg, beaten
- 380g plain flour (plus extra for dusting)

For the filling
- 100g butter
- 150g brown sugar, plus extra for sprinkling
- 2 tbsp ground cinnamon

These may take some time but they are oh so worth it. Sugar is vital to this recipe: it provides food for the yeast, which produces gases such as carbon dioxide in bubbles, causing the dough to rise. The soft brown sugar then melts perfectly into the butter and cinnamon in the filling, creating an overall deliciously doughy roll that you just can't get enough of.

Mix together the warm milk, yeast, sugar, salt, butter and egg. Make sure the milk isn't so hot that it kills the yeast! Mix in the flour and leave to one side to prove for an hour at room temperature.

Prepare the filling: melt the butter. Mix together the sugar and cinnamon. Line a large baking tray with baking paper.

Roll out the dough into a 30x45cm rectangle on a floured surface. Use as much flour as needed to ensure the dough doesn't stick. Brush generously with melted butter, all the way to the edges.

Sprinkle the cinnamon sugar on top, again spreading it all the way to the edges. Roll into a tight spiral, starting from the shorter end.

Slice into 12 pieces, placing each one cut-side down on the baking tray. Leave to prove for 30 minutes.

Preheat the oven to 160°C fan/180°C conventional/gas mark 4. Sprinkle with a little extra brown sugar and bake the rolls for 15–20 minutes, until golden brown on top.

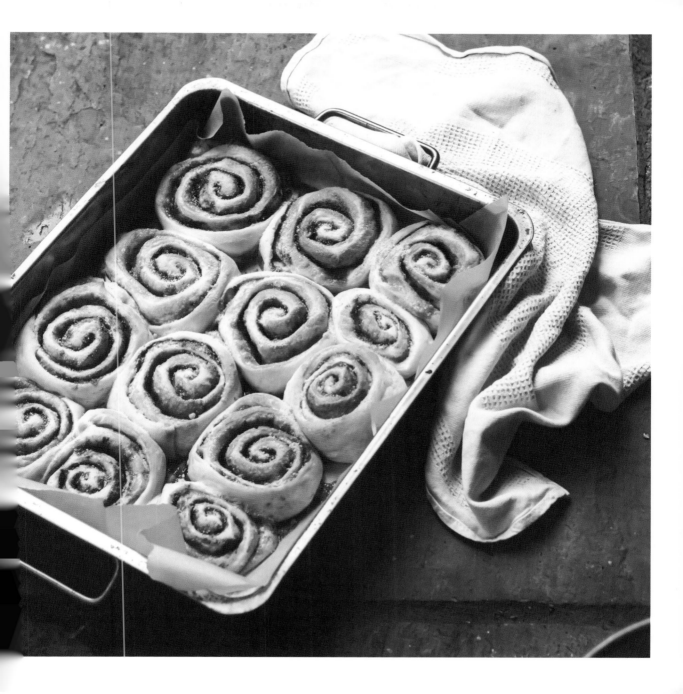

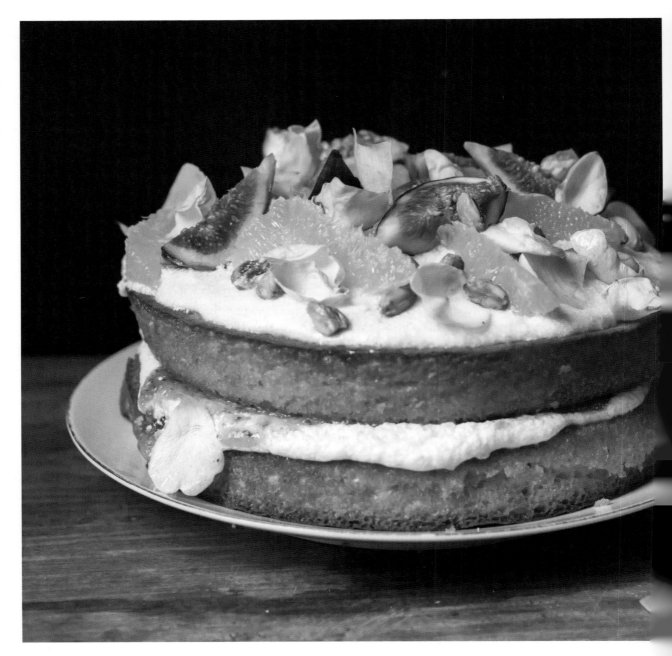

FIG & ORANGE CAKE

- 200g unsalted butter (room temperature), plus extra for greasing the tins
- 200g golden caster sugar
- 1 orange, zested and juiced
- 4 medium eggs, beaten
- 200g self-raising flour
- 1 tsp baking powder

For the buttercream
- 75g unsalted butter (softened, not melted)
- 250g icing sugar
- 1 orange, zested and 1 tbsp juice

For the fig paste
- 1 fresh fig
- 1 tbsp runny honey

To decorate
- Orange and fig segments
- Rose petals
- Shelled pistachios (optional)

You will need
- Two 20cm diameter tins

Figs are my favourite fruit, but on their own I just don't think they provide enough flavour to a cake. Pair them with orange and there you have perfection! This cake combines an orange sponge with fig paste, orange buttercream and plenty of figs to decorate.

Preheat the oven to 160°C fan/180°C conventional/gas mark 4. Mix together the cake ingredients, adding the flour and baking powder last and folding in carefully.

Put half the cake mixture in each tin and bake for around 25 minutes, until golden and an inserted toothpick comes out clean. In the meantime, mix together the buttercream ingredients and chill.

For the fig paste, blitz the ingredients together in a food processor and store at room temperature.

Leave the cakes to cool before taking them out of their tins. If not serving immediately, refrigerate the sponges and assemble just before serving.

To assemble, choose the half with the least attractive top, and place it upside down on a serving plate. Add a thin layer of buttercream, then the fig paste, then another thin layer of buttercream. Carefully place the other cake half on top, right-side up. Gently add the rest of the buttercream on top and decorate with orange and fig segments, rose petals and pistachios (if using).

LEMON VANILLA CHEESECAKE

SERVES 8

- 250g digestive biscuits
- 100g butter, plus extra for greasing
- 500g cream cheese
- 100g icing sugar
- 1 tsp vanilla bean paste or essence
- 1 lemon, zested, and 1 tbsp of juice
- 200ml double cream
- Fresh fruit such as figs, blueberries, raspberries and cherries, and sprigs of freash mint, for topping

You will need

- A loose-based tart tin approximately 20cm in diameter

I've tried many a raw, dairy-free cheesecake in my wellness days, and while cashews do give a creamy texture, I find they're incredibly dense and have nothing on the real deal. This is the real deal, and it needs icing sugar because its incredibly fine texture allows it to be easily incorporated into a smooth, light mixture without the need for baking.

Grease the tart tin with a little butter and place a circle of baking paper in the bottom.

Crush the biscuits in a bowl. Melt the butter and mix into the biscuits. Press this into the base of the tin and leave to set in the fridge for 30–60 minutes.

Mix together the cream cheese, icing sugar, vanilla and lemon zest and juice. Lightly whip the double cream and fold this into the mixture.

Scoop this on top of the biscuit base and smooth out right to the edges. Put this back into the fridge for another few hours.

Just before serving, decorate with any fresh fruit you desire. I've used figs, blueberries, raspberries and cherries topped with sprigs of fresh mint.

TIP This can be kept in the fridge for up to a week.

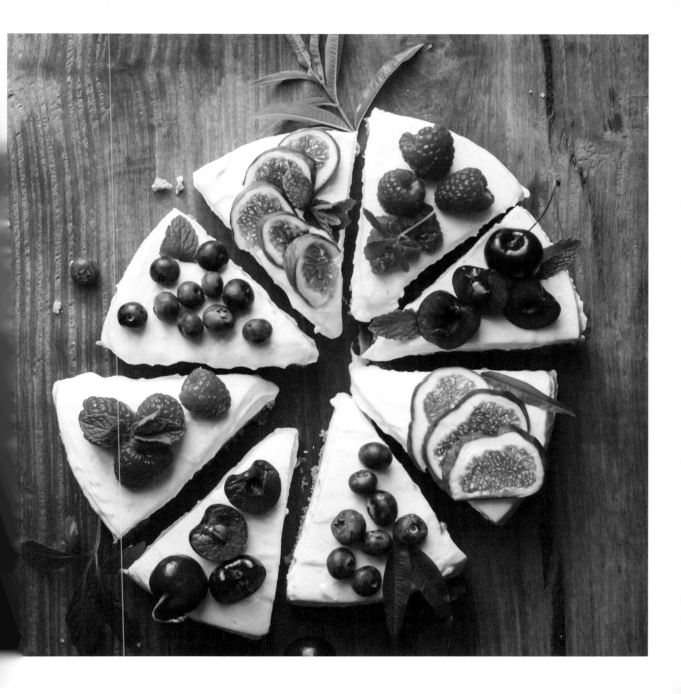

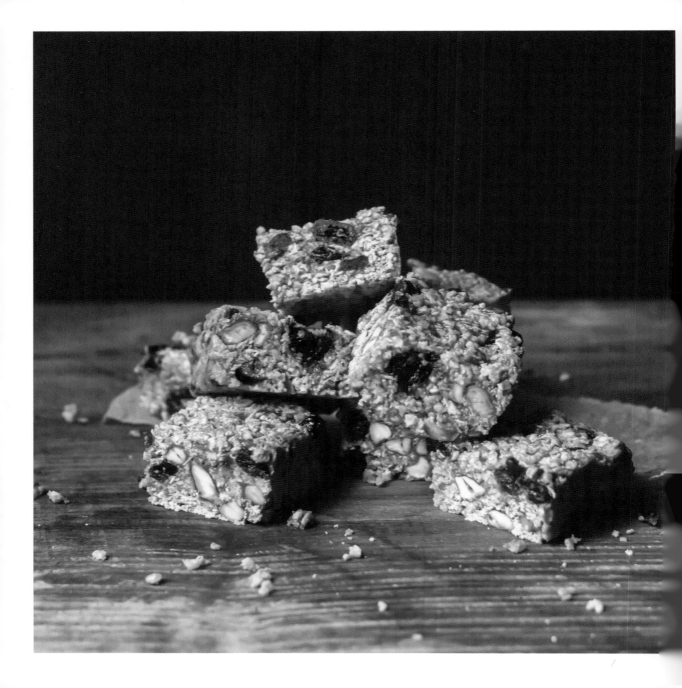

RAINBOW FLAPJACKS

MAKES 8 SQUARES

50g soft unsalted butter, plus extra for greasing
200g rolled oats
150g golden syrup
1 tsp cinnamon
1 medium egg, beaten
Pinch of salt
50g blueberries (fresh or frozen)
50g cranberries
50g shelled pistachios

You will need
- A 1.5 litre loaf tin
- Double up the recipe to make a traybake

When I was younger, I was chief brownie-maker, while my sister was in charge of flapjacks. Now I make them both! Personally, I find your standard flapjack slightly too sweet, so I like to add berries and nuts, which provide a more interesting texture and cut through the sweetness a little. However, no flapjack is complete without a decent dose of golden syrup – it's what makes it so deliciously gooey!

Preheat the oven to 180°C fan/200°C conventional/gas mark 6.

If the butter is too hard, soften it with brief bursts in the microwave.

Cream the butter with the oats, syrup, cinnamon, egg and salt. Gently stir in the blueberries, cranberries and pistachios.

Grease the loaf tin with a little butter and line with baking paper. Pour the mixture into the tin and press down firmly. Bake for around 20 minutes, until golden brown.

Leave to cool for 5 minutes before removing from the tin and cutting into 8 pieces.

 TIP These can be stored in an airtight container for up to 2 weeks.

PEAR & SALTED CARAMEL TART

SERVES 8-12

- 1 ready rolled shortcrust pastry sheet (320g)
- 50g granulated sugar
- 2 star anise
- 1 cinnamon stick
- 2 conference pears, peeled, halved and deseeded
- 375g caster sugar
- 100g golden syrup
- 100g butter
- 150ml double cream
- 1 tsp salt
- 50g chopped walnuts

You will need
- A loose-based tart tin approximately 25cm in diameter, greased

Proper caramel requires both a granulated and liquid sweetener. When they combine and work their magic you have the most delicious, thick, sweet mixture. Add the freshness of the pears and you have a winner.

Preheat the oven to 170°C fan/190°C conventional/gas mark 5.

Line the tart tin with the pastry, pressing gently into all corners and leaving some lightly overhanging. Prick the base with a fork and bake for 15 minutes. Leave to cool.

Bring 1 litre of water to the boil and add the granulated sugar, star anise and the cinnamon. Add the pears and poach for around 30 minutes, until a knife slides through easily. Remove and let cool.

Make the caramel: put 100ml of water into a pan along with the caster sugar and golden syrup. Simmer gently for 10–15 minutes, until the mixture is a deep brown caramel. Do not stir the mixture. Remove from the heat and add the butter, cream and salt. Stir until smooth, heating it slightly more if needed. Leave to cool slightly.

Once cool, place the pears on a board flat-side down and slice thinly.

Pour the caramel into the pastry case, fan out the pear slices, placing each fan gently on top of the caramel. Sprinkle the walnuts around the edges and in the centre. Chill for several hours, ideally overnight until set.

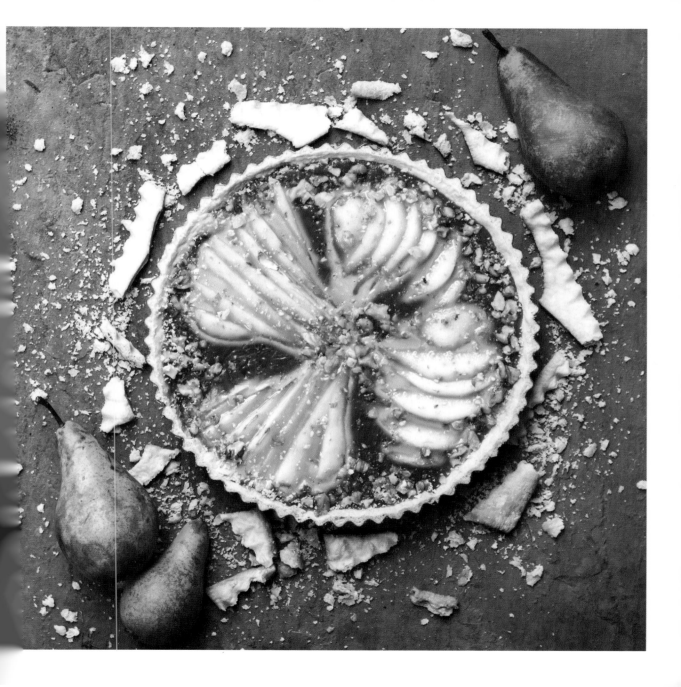

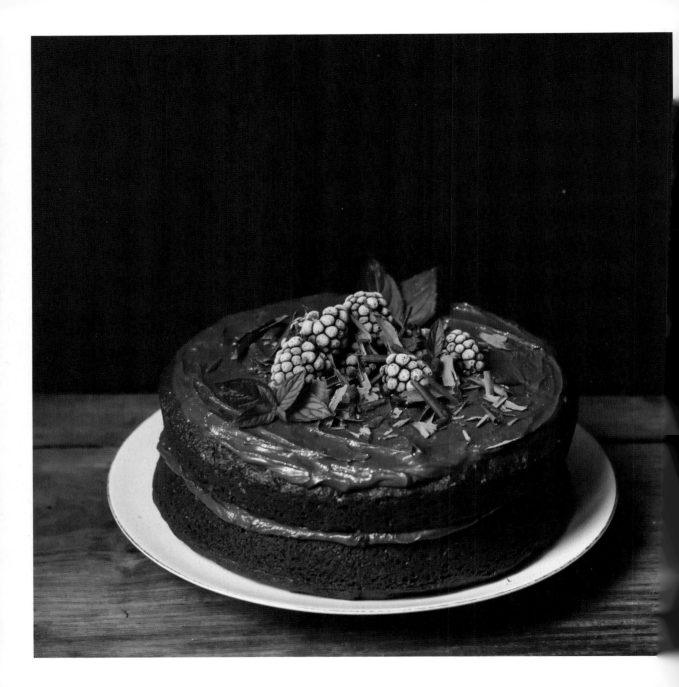

SUPER INDULGENT CHOCOLATE CAKE

SERVES 8

For the cake
- 150g butter
- 100g dark chocolate
- 1 tsp baking powder
- 30g cocoa powder
- 175g muscovado sugar
- 3 medium eggs, beaten
- 1 tsp vanilla bean paste or vanilla essence
- Pinch of salt
- 150g self-raising flour
- Chocolate shavings, to decorate

For the buttercream
- 150g dark chocolate
- 150g soft butter (not melted)
- 150g icing sugar

You will need
- Two 20cm springform cake tins, greased
- Electric mixer

No guilt-free bollocks here. This cake will satisfy all your chocolatey cravings and put a smile on your face. Don't waste your money buying raw cacao for this – you're going to bake it anyway! Muscovado sugar has a higher molasses content and has a slightly smoky aftertaste, which makes this chocolate cake taste even richer and more delicious.

Preheat the oven to 170°C fan/190°C conventional/gas mark 5.

Melt the butter and dark chocolate together in the microwave or in a heatproof bowl over a saucepan of gently simmering water. Add the rest of the cake ingredients and mix together, leaving the flour until last.

Divide the mixture evenly between the cake tins. Bake for 20–30 minutes, until an inserted toothpick comes out clean. Check every few minutes once it hits the 20-minute mark to avoid overbaking.

To make the buttercream, melt the dark chocolate in the microwave or in a heatproof bowl over a saucepan of gently simmering water. Use an electric mixer (if possible) to mix together the soft butter, melted chocolate and icing sugar until you have a thick buttercream.

When the cakes are ready, let cool completely. If you add the buttercream too soon it will split. Turn out the cakes, spread each with buttercream and place one on top of the other. Decorate with shaved chocolate and chill until 30 minutes before serving.

WHITE CHOCOLATE & RASPBERRY COOKIES

MAKES 10-12

- 7 tbsp olive oil
- 150g brown sugar
- 1 egg, beaten
- 1 tsp vanilla bean paste or vanilla essence
- Pinch of salt
- ½ tsp baking powder
- 180g plain flour
- 100g frozen raspberries
- 80-100g white chocolate chips

These cookies are dedicated to my sister Vivika, as it's her favourite flavour combination. I can definitely understand why. This recipe uses brown sugar as it helps provide the deliciously chewy texture.

Preheat the oven to 180°C fan/200°C conventional/gas mark 6.

In a bowl, mix together the olive oil, sugar, egg and vanilla bean paste or essence. Add the salt and baking powder and mix again. Add the flour, a little at a time, and mix until fully combined.

Chop the raspberries slightly – whole raspberries can make the cookies too soggy. Add the chocolate chips and raspberries to the cookie dough and stir.

Take tablespoons of the mixture and place them on a greased baking tray, spacing them out evenly. Gently form the dough into roughly round shapes. If any chocolate chips have come loose just press them on top.

Bake for 15-18 minutes, until the edges are just crispy but the middle is still soft.

Leave to cool for 15 minutes before touching or moving them.

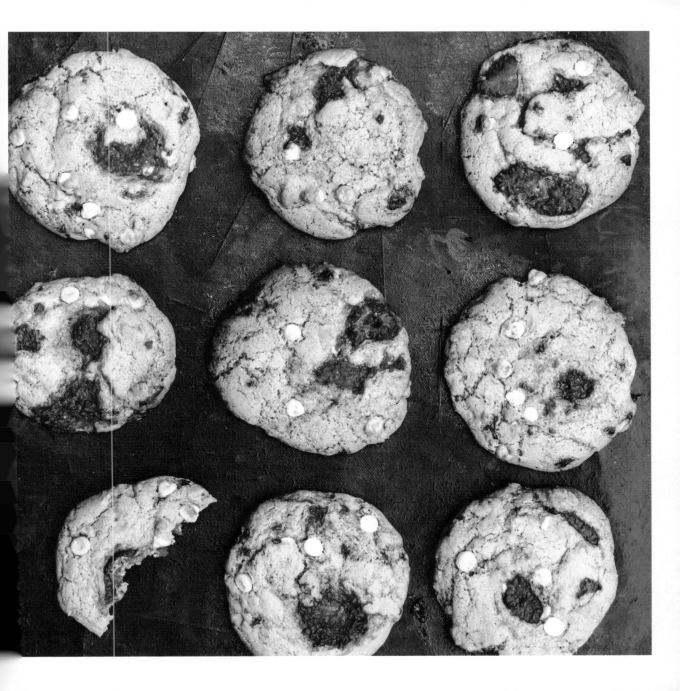

Enjoy your food

WHAT DOES IT REALLY TAKE TO BE HEALTHY?

Nutrition may seem like a complicated and confusing science, and with good reason – every day there seems to be a headline in the media saying, 'New study shows. . .'. Someone has even made a website dedicated to all the different foods the Daily Mail has claimed cure and cause cancer (some foods are even claimed to do both!). In general, the media are not great at reporting on science.

It's no wonder really that pseudoscience and myths like the ones discussed have been allowed to thrive. We like simple solutions, and we're much more comfortable with black and white, good and bad foods; eat this but don't eat that. It's the reason that we, as a general rule, don't follow government guidelines very well. The five-a-day message has been out there for ages now, and yet as a population we aren't meeting that. Telling us to eat more of something is far less effective than telling us to cut foods out, and that's where wellness thrives. Food packaging will proudly display everything it's 'free from' (soy, gluten, sugar, eggs, joy . . .) because what you don't eat is now more of a status symbol than what you do. If you look at any famous wellness blogger (or at least their 'food philosophy'), you'll find a list of foods that are deemed unacceptable, whether it's all animal products, gluten, legumes or grains. There's always something. Most commonly of all: processed foods, gluten and refined sugar. Hopefully by this point, you'll agree with me that it's just bollocks. But it works; people like it and people follow it and shout their success at having lost x kg and feeling amazing, because weight loss is almost always the goal. In the end, that's all wellness boils down to – an expensive, elitist weight-loss program under the guise of 'health' and 'lifestyle'. By cutting out foods like gluten and refined sugar, suddenly a whole host of highly palatable foods are off-limits, so obtaining enough calories isn't as easy as it was before, and weight comes off.

But with the rise of orthorexia and its link to the whole 'clean eating' movement, you could even go so far as to argue that wellness is simply a socially acceptable eating disorder.

WHY DO WE FALL FOR PSEUDOSCIENCE?

Aside from liking simple solutions – which pseudoscience tends to offer – rather than complex and more vague government guidelines, there are several other mistakes we make, which have cropped up throughout this book.

We often mistake correlation for causation. That is, we see two things that seem to be associated and assume one causes the other. Establishing causation is difficult enough as it is, but in nutrition, it's even harder due to the many confounding variables involved. Two examples already mentioned are a correlation between dairy consumption and rates of osteoporosis, and an association between cutting out gluten and feeling better. Although one is on a population level and the other at an individual level, neither shows that one thing causes another. You'll also find that the number of films Nicolas Cage appears in correlates with deaths by falling into a pool and drowning. That doesn't mean Nicolas Cage movies are causing people to drown, nor does it mean drowning people caused directors to cast Nicolas Cage in their movies.

Fearmongering tactics provide another explanation for why we fall for pseudoscience, and they often cause mass unnecessary dietary restriction. Telling someone not to eat something is one thing, but call it toxic and base your reasoning very (very) loosely on scientific principles we might vaguely remember from school, and you have a perfect recipe for scaring people out of eating foods they're actually probably fine eating. Naturally, wellness has thrived on this principle, and depending on where you look, either animal products, sugar or processed foods are killing us all, and the only way out is to stop eating them forever. Or, if it's not processed foods then its unpronounceable ingredients and scary chemicals in these foods that are the root of all evil. Being scared of eating particular foods is not the basis for a healthy relationship with food. If you're looking at a frozen ready meal and feel genuinely anxious and scared of eating it then something is wrong. It's one thing to simply not want to eat something, to make that choice, but quite another to feel such a negative emotional response to it.

What wellness fails to point out is that 'the dose makes the poison'. A documentary recently claimed that eating processed meats is as bad for you as plutonium, simply because they're both in the same category of carcinogens. But that's not how it works. You only need a small dose of plutonium for it to be carcinogenic, whereas eating 50g or more processed meats every day increases your chance of developing bowel cancer by 18%, equivalent to a 2.9% lifetime risk if you don't eat processed meat and 3.4% risk if you eat 50g each day [1]. They're just not comparable! Similarly, mercury is deemed a legitimate reason to avoid eating fish, but it's apparently fine when it's found in pink Himalayan salt [2]. (Side note: eating too much fish isn't recommended, hence the guidelines saying twice a week, but there's no need to cut fish out entirely when there are numerous nutritional benefits to eating it).

Desperation can also mean people fall for pseudoscience. We probably all know someone who has succumbed to wellness myths in a bid to cure themselves. When faced with a lifetime of pain, chronic conditions, degenerative illness or poor prognosis, of course you'd want to try anything to feel better. Even if it's completely batshit crazy. Anything you dismiss can be seen as not trying enough or not wanting it enough. And naturally, where there are desperate people, there are those willing to exploit them and take their money.

PIXIE TIP
A list of foods to cut out of your diets should always be a red flag, especially in books where the author has never even met you.

Which leads me nicely into my final theme . . . so-called 'experts' with no nutrition training trying to make money. While unqualified Instagrammers are the most obvious ones to avoid, I'm also including most media doctors as well, because doctors in the UK don't receive adequate nutrition training and certainly nothing close to registered nutritionists and dietitians. When someone is making a career out of writing controversial books and selling supplements on their website, and especially when what they're promoting doesn't fit the general scientific consensus, it's good to be sceptical. I'm not saying to automatically dismiss everything they're saying, but question whether there's compelling evidence that refutes their ideas. If someone has an agenda from the start (for example making a documentary or selling books that promote a single way of eating as the right way), then it's more likely that they will cherry-pick the evidence they want to present, rather than showing the overall picture.

There will almost always be a study that shows what you want to hear. Think of it this way: if you flip a coin ten times, there's a chance you might get ten heads in a row. If you only do this once, you might be forgiven for thinking the coin only has heads. But if you do this experiment hundreds of times, your results will eventually deviate towards 50% heads and 50% tails. The same concept applies towards scientific studies; there will be individual studies which show some crazy extreme results simply due to chance, but by doing similar experiments several times over and over and then analysing them all together in the form of a systematic review or meta-analysis, we can get an idea of the overall picture and use it to develop government guidelines on nutrition and public health. So please, next time you see a headline saying, 'New study shows that 'x' causes cancer' or something equally exciting or terrifying, remember that individual studies should always be taken with a pinch of salt.

Equally, this shows why anecdotes are not helpful. Only experiments that take hundreds or thousands of people (i.e. coin tosses) can give an accurate

If in doubt, it's always worth questioning someone and being sceptical of what you read.

picture. And again, this is why meta-analyses and government guidelines are more robust – more studies mean more people!

You could take this principle of cherry-picking and question whether I've done it, and you should. I've deliberately chosen to have a reference list in this book so that you can hopefully see that, where possible, I've referenced meta-analyses. And where there isn't enough data, I've tried to show both sides. Personally, I use artificial sweeteners in my coffee, but I've openly discussed the potential downsides of these. I also can't stand superfood powders, but have discussed the research showing that there might be some benefits to maca after all. I could have easily missed these out, but that wouldn't be very scientific of me.

In reality, the basics of good nutrition are extremely simple. Basically, everything in moderation. It sounds boring and that's why it's not popular

SO WHAT SHOULD WE BE EATING?

In reality, the basics of good nutrition are extremely simple: eat a varied, balanced diet, with a little bit of what you fancy. Basically, everything in moderation. It sounds boring and that's why it's not popular – it doesn't sell books, doesn't get TV ratings and doesn't inspire miracle cures or miracle foods. There is no quick or easy solution; it's not down to individual foods or nutrients, it's down to eating a variety of foods in the long term and not over-indulging in anything – even kale!

I like diagrams, so here's one I often use with my clients:

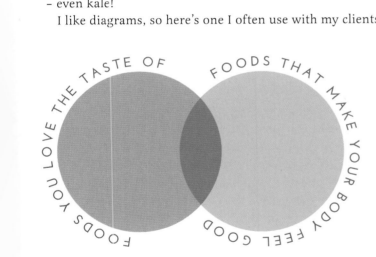

Ideally most of what you eat should fall in the middle – these are foods that make you feel happy as well as healthy, and are ideal to consume in large amounts, like your favourite vegetables. Then have a small amount of the foods that you love but which don't make you feel great in large amounts (like cake, for example), and don't bother with the ones you don't like the taste of, even if they're incredibly good for you like kale. Life's too short for that.

Ultimately, a healthy diet should not come at the expense of a healthy relationship with food –there's little point eating the healthiest diet in the world only to end up a one-hundred-year-old miserable sod. Because good health comes down to more than just eating well; it's having an overall healthy lifestyle including regular exercise, a good sleep pattern, the ability to cope with stress, genetics, good mental health, happiness and a balanced diet. Lack of sleep and high stress levels are often underplayed, when they can have a huge effect on wellbeing. Mental health is overlooked most of all, and socioeconomic factors barely even get a mention.

We too quickly forget that the populations who live the longest thrive on vastly varying diets, eat slowly and mindfully, and eat socially. They are proof that there is no one-size-fits-all solution to happiness and longevity. And this is why I will not tell you that there is one single way to eat, one single way to be healthy and won't give you a list of food rules to follow or foods to avoid. What I can give you is permission to eat foods that make you happy, and to not give a shit about what others think. Eat that cake, but also eat those vegetables, too. And don't confuse the two. Vegetables masquerading as cake probably won't satisfy you in the same way as the real deal would, so you're likely to end up overeating those sweet potato brownies, whereas you'd probably be happy with just the one real-deal brownie. So, enjoy your vegetables and enjoy your cake, just maybe not at the same time. And if you're that person who turns their nose up at that person eating a sausage roll on the train, stop and think for a second. What gives you the right to judge that person for their choice? You know nothing about them, including what else they may have done or eaten that day. You have no idea if this is a one-off or a regular decision they make. Don't judge. Hope that they're happy with their choice and be happy for them.

Life's too short to eat foods you don't like, no matter how 'healthy' they are.

I won't give you food rules, because I don't believe they are generally very helpful, but I can offer some general guidance on what constitutes a healthy diet.

• Eat a wide variety of foods.
• Don't completely avoid foods that make you happy.
• Don't completely sacrifice your social life only to eat a boring salad alone at home.
• If the way you eat doesn't make you happy, then change it up.

Vague, right? And no exclusions? There's a reason for that. The only foods you need to avoid are ones you're allergic to, ones that have gone-off, and ones that you don't like the taste of. Yet even within that there are exceptions: you might be partly lactose intolerant but still enjoy a cake someone made for you with love and butter, some foods are supposed to be gone-off, like cheese, and it's always worth giving foods you dislike another go at some point.

BECOME A BS DETECTOR

I don't want you to have to always rely on others to tell you what is good science and what's a load of nutribollocks. It's good to have the tools to do this yourself. Of course, a science degree is always the best option as you learn to analyse and interpret scientific evidence, and spend many an hour slaving over statistics. But this isn't realistic for everyone. Thanks to the internet, a basic level of scientific literacy among the general population has never been more important. It empowers you to critically analyse and evaluate statements, headlines and evidence that's thrown your way, and it stops you from being duped by snake-oil salesmen or women and dubious healthcare professionals claiming to cure the incurable. It could save you time, money and unnecessary anxiety around food. In an extreme situation, it could even save your life.

Without further ado, here are my top ten warning signs to help you detect nutribollocks online:

1. ONE SINGLE ANSWER TO ALL PROBLEMS, REGARDLESS OF CAUSE.
2. ONE-SIZE-FITS-ALL APPROACH TO EATING AND LIVING.
3. 'MIRACLE' OR 'SUPER' FOODS, WITH NO EVIDENCE TO SUPPORT THEM.
4. RELIANCE ON (UNPROVED) ANCIENT WISDOMS.
5. RELIANCE ON CONSPIRACY THEORIES.
6. COMPLETE REJECTION OF ANY EVIDENCE THAT DOESN'T SUPPORT THE ARGUMENT (CHERRY-PICKING STUDIES).
7. RELIANCE ON ANECDOTAL EVIDENCE.
8. TELLING YOU YOUR BODY IS FULL OF TOXINS, FOLLOWED BY HOW TO 'DETOXIFY' IT.
9. NATURALISTIC FALLACY ('NATURAL IS ALWAYS BETTER').
10. FEARMONGERING ABOUT FOODS AND PARTICULAR INGREDIENTS.

If you see any of these things, be sceptical. Even if it forces you to challenge your ideas around food. Especially if it forces you to challenge your ideas, in fact. This doesn't mean that you can immediately discard anything that uses these methods, or that you should make an immediate assumption that it's all nutribollocks, just that you need to critically analyse the information that is presented to you. Ideally, you should always be sceptical of any nutrition information you're presented with, and question every source, but these ten strategies should send your bullshit detectors tingling.

FINAL THOUGHTS...

If you have the money to spend on this book, you are probably in a wonderful position of privilege; you're in a place where you have the luxury of concerning yourself with the finer details of what and how to eat, as opposed to simply trying to ward off starvation. And with the rise of orthorexia, many of us could do with chilling out a bit about what we eat, ditching the diet rules and deprivation mentality and placing enjoyment of food on a par with health, at the very least.

I want you to put this book down having learnt something new, to be less scared of foods and to think more sceptically about what you read online. But most of all, I want you to leave with an appreciation of just how amazing food is, and how enjoying food is a key part of living a healthy, happy life. Food is a wonderful thing. Food brings people together, we use food to mark special occasions and a single smell can instantly bring on waves of nostalgia. We eat food every day – you can't escape it – and because of that, our relationship with food is vitally important. We should have a happy relationship with what we eat, not one where food makes us anxious and scared.

Go forth, wellness rebel!

References

INTRO/EAT CLEAN [1] www.bhf.org.uk/heart-matters- magazine/medical/familial-hypercholesterolaemia

INTRO/EAT REAL FOOD [1] Nordmann, A., Nordmann, A., Briel, M., Keller, U., Yancy, W., Brehm, B. and Bucher, H. (2006). Effects of low-carbohydrate vs low-fat diets on weight loss and cardiovascular risk factors. *Archives of Internal Medicine*, 166(3), p.285.
[2] Berg JM, Tymoczko JL, Stryer L. Biochemistry. 5th edition. New York: W H Freeman; 2002. Section 22.1, Triacylglycerols are highly concentrated energy stores.
[3] Wong, J., de Souza, R., Kendall, C., Emam, A. and Jenkins, D. (2006). Colonic health: fermentation and short chain fatty acids. *Journal of Clinical Gastroenterology*, 40(3), pp.235–243.
[4] Kim, Y. and Je, Y. (2016). Dietary fibre intake and mortality from cardiovascular disease and all cancers: A meta-analysis of prospective cohort studies. *Archives of Cardiovascular Diseases*, 109(1), pp.39–54.
[5] Park, Y., Subar, A., Hollenbeck, A. and Schatzkin, A. (2011). Dietary fiber intake and mortality in the NIH-AARP diet and health study. *Archives of Internal Medicine*, 171(12).
[6] Dietary fibre and incidence of type 2 diabetes in eight European countries: the EPIC-InterAct Study and a meta-analysis of prospective studies. (2015). *Diabetologia*, 58(7), pp.1394–1408.
[7] Nhs.uk. (2017). *Constipation – NHS Choices*. [online] www.nhs.uk/Conditions/Constipation/Pages/Introduction.aspx [Accessed 31 Aug. 2017].
[8] Puhl, R. and Heuer, C. (2009). The stigma of obesity: a review and update. *Obesity*, 17(5), pp.941–964.

GLUTEN [1] Moore, M.M., Schober, T.J., Dockery, P. and Arendt, E.K., 2004. Textural comparisons of gluten-free and wheat-based doughs, batters, and breads. *Cereal Chemistry*, 81(5), pp.567–575.
[2] Nhs.uk. (2017). *Coeliac disease – NHS Choices*. [online] www.nhs.uk/Conditions/Coeliac-disease/Pages/Introduction.aspx [Accessed 31 Aug. 2017].
[3] Lundin, K.E. and Alaedini, A., 2012. Non-celiac gluten sensitivity. *Gastrointestinal Endoscopy Clinics of North America*, 22(4), pp.723–734.
[4] Biesiekierski, J.R., Peters, S.L., Newnham, E.D., Rosella, O., Muir, J.G. and Gibson, P.R., 2013. No effects of gluten in patients with self-reported non-celiac gluten sensitivity after dietary reduction of fermentable, poorly absorbed, short-chain carbohydrates. *Gastroenterology*, 145(2), pp.320–328.
[5] Halmos, E.P., Christophersen, C.T., Bird, A.R., Shepherd, S.J., Gibson, P.R. and Muir, J.G., 2014. Diets that differ in their FODMAP content alter the colonic luminal microenvironment. *Gut*, pp.gutjnl-2014.
[6] Thompson, T., 2000. Folate, iron, and dietary fiber contents of the gluten-free diet. *Journal of the American Dietetic Association*, 100(11), pp.1389–1396.
[7] Mariani, P., Viti, M.G., Montouri, M., La Vecchia, A., Cipolletta, E., Calvani, L. and Bonamico, M., 1998. The gluten-free diet: a nutritional risk factor for adolescents with celiac disease?. *Journal of Pediatric Gastroenterology and Nutrition*, 27(5), pp.519–523.
[8] Saturni, L., Ferretti, G. and Bacchetti, T.,
2010. The gluten-free diet: safety and nutritional quality. *Nutrients*, 2(1), pp.16–34.
[9] Alvarez-Jubete, L., Arendt, E.K. and Gallagher, E., 2010. Nutritive value of pseudocereals and their increasing use as functional gluten-free ingredients. *Trends in Food Science & Technology*, 21(2), pp.106–113.
[10] De Palma, G., Nadal, I., Collado, M.C. and Sanz, Y., 2009. Effects of a gluten-free diet on gut microbiota and immune function in healthy adult human subjects. *British Journal of Nutrition*, 102(8), pp.1154–1160.
[11] Singh, J. and Whelan, K., 2011. Limited availability and higher cost of gluten-free foods. *Journal of Human Nutrition and Dietetics*, 24(5), pp.479–486.

DETOX [1] Vanin, J. and Saylor, K. (1989). Laxative abuse: a hazardous habit for weight control. *Journal of American College Health*, 37(5), pp.227–230.
[2] Dordoni, B., Willson, R., Thompson, R. and Williams, R. (1973). Reduction of absorption of paracetamol by activated charcoal and cholestyramine: a possible therapeutic measure. *BMJ*, 3(5871), pp.86–87.
[3] Hultén, B., Heath, A., Mellstrand, T. and Hedner, T. (1986). Does alcohol absorb to activated charcoal?. *Human Toxicology*, 5(3), pp.211–212.
[4] Kadakal, Ç., Poyrazoglu, E., Artik, N. And Nas, S. (2004). Effect of activated charcoal on water-soluble vitamin content of apple Juice. *Journal of Food Quality*, 27(2), pp.171–180.
[5] Dangour, A., Lock, K., Hayter, A., Aikenhead, A., Allen, E. and Uauy, R. (2010). Nutrition-related health effects of organic foods: a systematic review. *American Journal of Clinical Nutrition*, 92(1), pp.203–210.

[6] Smith-Spangler, C., Brandeau, M., Hunter, G., Bavinger, J., Pearson, M., Eschbach, P., Sundaram, V., Liu, H., Schirmer, P., Stave, C., Olkin, I. and Bravata, D. (2012). Are organic foods safer or healthier than conventional alternatives?. *Annals of Internal Medicine*, 157(5), p.348.

[7] Bergmann, M. et al. (2013). The association of pattern of lifetime alcohol use and cause of death in the European Prospective Investigation into Cancer and Nutrition (EPIC) study. *International Journal of Epidemiology*, 42(6), pp.1772–1790.

F A T S [1] Manninen, V., Tenkanen, L., Koskinen, P., Huttunen, J., Manttari, M., Heinonen, O. and Frick, M. (1992). Joint effects of serum triglyceride and LDL cholesterol and HDL cholesterol concentrations on coronary heart disease risk in the Helsinki Heart Study. Implications for treatment. *Circulation*, 85(1), pp.37–45.

[2] Fernandez, M.L. and West, K.L., 2005. Mechanisms by which dietary fatty acids modulate plasma Lipids1. *The Journal of Nutrition*, 135(9), pp.2075–2078.

[3] Mozaffarian, D., Katan, M.B., Ascherio, A., Stampfer, M.J. and Willett, W.C., 2006. Trans fatty acids and cardiovascular disease. *New England Journal of Medicine*, 354(15), pp.1601–1613.

[4] Hooper, L., Martin, N., Abdelhamid, A. and Davey Smith, G., 2015. Reduction in saturated fat intake for cardiovascular disease. *The Cochrane Library*.

[5] Chen, M., Li, Y., Sun, Q., Pan, A., Manson, J.E., Rexrode, K.M., Willett, W.C., Rimm, E.B. and Hu, F.B., 2016. Dairy fat and risk of cardiovascular disease in 3 cohorts of US adults. *The American Journal of Clinical Nutrition*, 104(5), pp.1209–1217.

[6] Shin, J.Y., Xun, P., Nakamura, Y. and He, K., 2013. Egg consumption in relation to risk of cardiovascular disease and diabetes: a systematic review and meta-analysis. *The American Journal of Clinical Nutrition*, pp.ajcn-051318.

[7] Santos, F.L., Esteves, S.S., da Costa Pereira, A., Yancy Jr, W.S. and Nunes, J.P.L., 2012. Systematic review and meta-analysis of clinical trials of the effects of low carbohydrate diets on cardiovascular risk factors. *Obesity Reviews*, 13(11), pp.1048–1066.

[8] Eyres, L., Eyres, M.F., Chisholm, A. and Brown, R.C., 2016. Coconut oil consumption and cardiovascular risk factors in humans. *Nutrition Reviews*, 74(4), pp.267–280.

[9] Marten, B., Pfeuffer, M. and Schrezenmeir, J., 2006. Medium-chain triglycerides. *International Dairy Journal*, 16(11), pp.1374–1382.

[10] Stanley, J.C., Elsom, R.L., Calder, P.C., Griffin, B.A., Harris, W.S., Jebb, S.A., Lovegrove, J.A., Moore, C.S., Riemersma, R.A. and Sanders, T.A., 2007. UK Food Standards Agency Workshop Report: the effects of the dietary n-6: n-3 fatty acid ratio on cardiovascular health. *British Journal of Nutrition*, 98(6), pp.1305–1310.

[11] Lin, L., Allemekinders, H., Dansby, A., Campbell, L., Durance-Tod, S., Berger, A. and Jones, P.J., 2013. Evidence of health benefits of canola oil. *Nutrition Reviews*, 71(6), pp.370–385.

[12] Gov.uk. (2017). *Family Food Statistics - GOV.UK*. [online] Available at: www.gov.uk/government/collections/family-food- statistics [Accessed 31 Aug. 2017].

[13] Rippe, J.M. and Angelopoulos, T.J., 2015. Sugars and health controversies: what does the science say?. *Advances in Nutrition: An International Review Journal*, 6(4), pp.493S–503S.

S U P E R F O O D S [1] Hemilä, H. and Chalker, E., 2013. Vitamin C for preventing and treating the common cold. *The Cochrane Library*.

[2] Karlowski, T.R., Chalmers, T.C., Frenkel, L.D., Kapikian, A.Z., Lewis, T.L. and Lynch, J.M., 1975. Ascorbic acid for the common cold: a prophylactic and therapeutic trial. *Jama*, 231(10), pp.1038–1042.

[3] Creagan, E.T., Moertel, C.G., O'Fallon, J.R., Schutt, A.J., O'Connell, M.J., Rubin, J. and Frytak, S., 1979. Failure of high-dose vitamin C (ascorbic acid) therapy to benefit patients with advanced cancer: a controlled trial. *New England Journal of Medicine*, 301(13), pp.687–690.

[4] Gonzales, G.F., Cordova, A., Vega, K., Chung, A., Villena, A. and Góñez, C., 2003. Effect of Lepidium meyenii (Maca), a root with aphrodisiac and fertility-enhancing properties, on serum reproductive hormone levels in adult healthy men. *Journal of Endocrinology*, 176(1), pp.163–168.

[5] Gonzales, G.F., Cordova, A., Vega, K., Chung, A., Villena, A., Góñez, C. and Castillo, S., 2002. Effect of Lepidium meyenii (Maca) on sexual desire and its absent relationship with serum testosterone levels in adult healthy men. *aNDROLOGia*, 34(6), pp.367–372.

[6] Dording, C.M., Fisher, L., Papakostas, G., Farabaugh, A., Sonawalla, S., Fava, M. and Mischoulon, D., 2008. A double-blind, randomized, pilot dose-finding study of maca root (L. Meyenii) for the Management of SSRI-Induced Sexual Dysfunction. *CNS Neuroscience & Therapeutics*, 14(3), pp.182–191.

[7] Lee, M.S., Shin, B.C., Yang, E.J., Lim, H.J.

and Ernst, E., 2011. Maca (Lepidium meyenii) for treatment of menopausal symptoms: a systematic review. *Maturitas*, 70(3), pp.227–233. www.ncbi.nlm.nih.gov/pubmed/21840656

[8] McCarron, P., Logan, A.C., Giddings, S.D. and Quilliam, M.A., 2014. Analysis of ß- N-methylamino- L-alanine (BMAA) in spirulina-containing supplements by liquid chromatography-tandem mass spectrometry. *Aquatic Biosystems*, 10(1), p.5.

[9] Glover, W., Baker, T.C., Murch, S.J. and Brown, P., 2015. Determination of ß-N- methylamino-L- alanine, N-(2- aminoethyl) glycine, and 2, 4-diaminobutyric acid in food products containing cyanobacteria by ultra-performance liquid chromatography and tandem mass spectrometry: single-laboratory validation. *Journal of AOAC International*, 98(6), pp.1559–1565.

[10] Rellán, S., Osswald, J., Saker, M., Gago-Martinez, A. and Vasconcelos, V., 2009. First detection of anatoxin-a in human and animal dietary supplements containing cyanobacteria. *Food and Chemical Toxicology*, 47(9), pp.2189–2195.

[11] Pablo, J., Banack, S.A., Cox, P.A., Johnson, T.E., Papapetropoulos, S., Bradley, W.G., Buck, A. and Mash, D.C., 2009. Cyanobacterial neurotoxin BMAA in ALS and Alzheimer's disease. *Acta Neurologica Scandinavica*, 120(4), pp.216–225.

[12] Watanabe, F., 2007. Vitamin B12 sources and bioavailability. *Experimental Biology and Medicine*, 232(10), pp.1266–1274.

[13] Bradbury, K.E., Appleby, P.N. and Key, T.J., 2014. Fruit, vegetable, and fiber intake in relation to cancer risk: findings from the European Prospective Investigation into Cancer and Nutrition (EPIC). *The American Journal of Clinical Nutrition*, 100(Supplement 1), pp.394S–398S.

[14] Peto, R., Doll, R., Buckley, J.D. and Sporn, M.B., 1981. Can dietary beta-carotene materially reduce human cancer rates? *Nature*, 290(5803), pp.201–208.

[15] Chen, G.C., Lu, D.B., Pang, Z. and Liu, Q.F., 2013. Vitamin C intake, circulating vitamin C and risk of stroke: a meta-analysis of prospective studies. *Journal of the American Heart Association*, 2(6), p.e000329.www.ncbi.nlm.nih.gov/pmc/articles/PMC3886767/

[16] Bjelakovic, G., Nikolova, D., Gluud, L.L., Simonetti, R.G. and Gluud, C., 2007. Mortality in randomized trials of antioxidant supplements for primary and secondary prevention: systematic review and meta-analysis. *Jama*, 297(8), pp.842–857.

[17] Ding, M., Satija, A., Bhupathiraju, S.N., Hu, Y., Sun, Q., Han, J., Lopez-Garcia, E., Willett, W., van Dam, R.M. and Hu, F.B., 2015. Association of coffee consumption with total and cause-specific mortality in three large prospective cohorts. *Circulation*, pp.CIRCULATIONAHA-115.

ALKALINE [1] Darling, A.L., Millward, D.J., Torgerson, D.J., Hewitt, C.E. and Lanham-New, S.A., 2009. Dietary protein and bone health: a systematic review and meta-analysis. *The American Journal of Clinical Nutrition*, 90(6), pp.1674–1692.

[2] Kerstetter, J.E., O'brien, K.O., Caseria, D.M., Wall, D.E. and Insogna, K.L., 2005. The impact of dietary protein on calcium absorption and kinetic measures of bone turnover in women. *The Journal of Clinical Endocrinology & Metabolism*, 90(1), pp.26–31.

[3] Fenton, T.R., Lyon, A.W., Eliasziw, M., Tough, S.C. and Hanley, D.A., 2009. Meta-analysis of the effect of the acid-ash

hypothesis of osteoporosis on calcium balance. *Journal of Bone and Mineral Research*, 24(11), pp.1835–1840.

[4] Fenton, T.R., Lyon, A.W., Eliasziw, M., Tough, S.C. and Hanley, D.A., 2009. Phosphate decreases urine calcium and increases calcium balance: a meta-analysis of the osteoporosis acid-ash diet hypothesis. *Nutrition Journal*, 8(1), p.41.

[5] Schwalfenberg, G.K., 2012. The alkaline diet: is there evidence that an alkaline pH diet benefits health?. *Journal of Environmental and Public Health*, 2012.

[6] Adeva, M.M. and Souto, G., 2011. Diet-induced metabolic acidosis. *Clinical Nutrition*, 30(4), pp.416–421.

[7] The National Diet and Nutrition Survey, 2014. www.gov.uk/government/statistics/national-diet-and-nutrition-survey-results-from-years-1-to-4-combined-of-the-rolling-programme-for-2008-and-2009-to-2011-and-2012

RAW FOODS [1] Hobbs, S.H., 2005. Attitudes, practices, and beliefs of individuals consuming a raw foods diet. *Explore: The Journal of Science and Healing*, 1(4), pp.272–277.

[2] Rickman, J.C., Barrett, D.M. and Bruhn, C.M., 2007. Nutritional comparison of fresh, frozen and canned fruits and vegetables. Part 1. Vitamins C and B and phenolic compounds. *Journal of the Science of Food and Agriculture*, 87(6), pp.930–944.

[3] Rickman, J.C., Bruhn, C.M. and Barrett, D.M., 2007. Nutritional comparison of fresh, frozen, and canned fruits and vegetables II. Vitamin A and carotenoids, vitamin E, minerals and fiber. *Journal of the Science of Food and Agriculture*, 87(7), pp.1185–1196.

[4] Chai, W. and Liebman, M., 2005. Effect

of different cooking methods on vegetable oxalate content. *Journal of Agricultural and Food Chemistry*, 53(8), pp.3027-3030.

[5] Hotz, C. and Gibson, R.S., 2007. Traditional food-processing and preparation practices to enhance the bioavailability of micronutrients in plant-based diets. *The Journal of Nutrition*, 137(4), pp.1097-1100.

[6] Urbano, G., Lopez-Jurado, M., Aranda, P., Vidal-Valverde, C., Tenorio, E. and Porres, J., 2000. The role of phytic acid in legumes: antinutrient or beneficial function?. *Journal of Physiology and Biochemistry*, 56(3), pp.283-294.

[7] Jiménez-Monreal, A.M., García-Diz, L., Martínez-Tomé, M., Mariscal, M.M.M.A. and Murcia, M.A., 2009. Influence of cooking methods on antioxidant activity of vegetables. *Journal of Food Science*, 74(3).

[8] Koebnick, C., Garcia, A.L., Dagnelie, P.C., Strassner, C., Lindemans, J., Katz, N., Leitzmann, C. and Hoffmann, I., 2005. Long-term consumption of a raw food diet is associated with favorable serum LDL cholesterol and triglycerides but also with elevated plasma homocysteine and low serum HDL cholesterol in humans. *The Journal of Nutrition*, 135(10), pp.2372-2378.

[9] Pawlak, R., Parrott, S.J., Raj, S., Cullum-Dugan, D. and Lucus, D., 2013. How prevalent is vitamin B12 deficiency among vegetarians?. *Nutrition Reviews*, 71(2), pp.110-117.

[10] Fontana, L., Shew, J.L., Holloszy, J.O. and Villareal, D.T., 2005. Low bone mass in subjects on a long-term raw vegetarian diet. *Archives of Internal Medicine*, 165(6), pp.684-689.

[11] Koebnick, C., Strassner, C., Hoffmann, I. and Leitzmann, C., 1999. Consequences of a long-term raw food diet on body weight and menstruation: results of a questionnaire survey. *Annals of Nutrition and Metabolism*, 43(2), pp.69-79.

[12] People dying in the care of raw foodies: www.mbp.state.md.us/pages/sanctions. html www.vegsource.com/talk/raw/messages/100032793.html

SUGAR [1] Carbohydrates, SACN., 2015. Health report. England PH, editor. www.gov.uk/government/publications/sacn-carbohydrates-and-health-report

[2] Aguilar, F., Charrondiere, U.R., Dusemund, B., Galtier, P., Gilbert, J. and Gott, D.M., 2010. Scientific opinion on the safety of steviol glycosides for the proposed uses as a food additive. *EFSA J*, 8, p.1537.

[3] Europäische Kommission Scientific Committee on Food, 2000. *Opinion of the Scientific Committee on Food on Sucralose*. www.ec.europa.eu/food/sites/food/files/safety/docs/sci-com_scf_out68_en.pdf

[4] Panel, E.A., 2013. Scientific opinion on the re-evaluation of aspartame (E 951) as a food additive. *EFSA J*, 11. www.onlinelibrary.wiley.com/doi/10.2903/j.efsa.2013.3496/abstract

[5] Lim, U., Subar, A.F., Mouw, T., Hartge, P., Morton, L.M., Stolzenberg-Solomon, R., Campbell, D., Hollenbeck, A.R. and Schatzkin, A., 2006. Consumption of aspartame-containing beverages and incidence of hematopoietic and brainmalignancies. *Cancer Epidemiology and Prevention Biomarkers*, 15(9), pp.1654-1659.

[6] Miller, P.E. and Perez, V., 2014. Low-calorie sweeteners and body weight and composition: a meta-analysis of randomized controlled trials and prospective cohort studies. *The American Journal of Clinical Nutrition*, 100(3), pp.765-777.

[7] Suez, J., Korem, T., Zeevi, D., Zilberman-Schapira, G., Thaiss, C.A., Maza, O., Israeli, D., Zmora, N., Gilad, S., Weinberger, A. and Kuperman, Y., 2014. Artificial sweeteners induce glucose intolerance by altering the gut microbiota. *Nature*, 514(7521), pp.181-186.

[8] Bellisle, F., 2015. Intense sweeteners, appetite for the sweet taste, and relationship to weight management. *Current Obesity Reports*, 4(1), pp.106-110.www.link.springer.com/article/10.1007/s13679-014-0133-8

[9] Meni, A.C.S., Swithers, S.E. and Rother, K.I., 2015. Positive association between artificially sweetened beverage consumption and incidence of diabetes. *Diabetologia*, 58(10), pp.2455-2456.

[10] Avena, N.M., Rada, P. and Hoebel, B.G., 2008. Evidence for sugar addiction: behavioral and neurochemical effects of intermittent, excessive sugar intake. *Neuroscience & Biobehavioral Reviews*, 32(1), pp.20-39.

[11] Lenoir, M., Serre, F., Cantin, L. and Ahmed, S.H., 2007. Intense sweetness surpasses cocaine reward. *PloS one*, 2(8), p.e698. www.journals.plos.org/plosone/article?id=10.1371/journal.pone.0000698

[12] Westwater, M.L., Fletcher, P.C. and Ziauddeen, H., 2016. Sugar addiction: the state of the science. *European Journal of Nutrition*, 55(2), pp.55-69.

CONCLUSION / ENJOY YOUR FOOD [1] Carcinogenicity of consumption of red and processed meat. www.thelancet.com/journals/lanonc/article/PIIS1470-2045(15)00444-1/fulltext

[2] Minerals in Himalayan Pink Salt: Spectral Analysis. www.themeadow.com/pages/minerals-in- himalayan-pink- salt-spectral- analysis

Index